To Steve,
Merry Christmas + best wishes
for a Happy New Year,

Robert Mudd

Handbook for the ORTHOPAEDIC ASSISTANT

Handbook for the
ORTHOPAEDIC ASSISTANT

F. Richard Schneider, M.D.

Clinical Coordinator, Orthopaedic Assistant's Program, City College of San Francisco;
Assistant Clinical Professor in Orthopaedics,
University of California School of Medicine, San Francisco;
Member of Subcommittee on the Training of the Orthopaedic Assistant,
American Academy of Orthopaedic Surgery

With 177 illustrations by
ROGER STRINGHAM

SAINT LOUIS

The C. V. Mosby Company

1972

PREFACE

Orthopaedics is that branch of medicine that deals with the prevention, diagnosis, and treatment of injuries to and diseases of the musculoskeletal system. This specialty lends itself particularly well to a team approach in the delivery of health care services, for certain observations required to establish the diagnosis and various tasks performed in the treatment do not require the broad educational background of the orthopaedic surgeon. These aspects may be delegated to an orthopaedic assistant. However, for this health personnel to be effective, he must be familiar with relevant didactic material and perform technical skills with expertise. This handbook was written toward this goal.

Most informational texts now available to medical students in the specialty of orthopaedic surgery are of two general types. The first describes bone and joint trauma in a geographic and systematic fashion. These texts give an overview of the diagnostic problems. Statements regarding treatment are usually brief and contained in such comments as "reduction by skeletal traction," "immobilization by a Velpeau dressing," or "the application of a plaster cast." The principles of cast immobilization may be mentioned; however, the technical aspects of plaster of Paris application are left for the student to learn in an on-the-job situation. The principles of traction in the treatment of trauma are similarly described.

The second type of textbook presents all aspects of this medical specialty including congenital anomalies, developmental abnormalities, infections, tumors of bone and other connective tissues, as well as an introduction into traumatology. The emphasis is placed on the recognition of disease entities and only secondarily on treatment. The text describes the pathology of congenital dislocation of the hip and the physical findings pertinent to the diagnosis. Alternatives in treatment of this condition are suggested by such statements as "gentle abduction traction," "closed reduction and the application of a hip spica cast," or "open reduction." Patients in specific casts or traction are illustrated, but without information relative to the application of the apparatus.

The medical student's brief exposure to orthopaedic surgery is not sufficient to allow him to formulate clinically sound decisions regarding treatment in any

v

specific case. If judgments concerning treatments are not to be made, the tools of management, namely the techniques of plaster of Paris and traction, are therefore irrelevant and not included in such a text.

The orthopaedic assistant working under the direction of the orthopaedic surgeon utilizes these techniques and must understand their inherent dangers. He should have a sufficient knowledge of orthopaedics to make certain judgments and translate them into specific appropriate actions. This textbook emphasizes basic principles and techniques primarily in the management of trauma, but these may be readily applied to other areas. Specific fractures or dislocations are not covered, except by example. Esoteric pathologic conditions have been deliberately excluded, as the acquisition of this knowledge is not relevant. The assistant is an extension of the orthopaedic surgeon and must be given a special sense for the specialty. To communicate with the orthopaedic surgeon, he requires the accumulation of a new vocabulary. To deal with patients, he must develop concern and respect for people who are ill. An effort is made to combine pertinent information with the necessary attitudes.

The chapters dealing with history taking and the physical examination should be considered only the foundation upon which the assistant may build as he develops his skills. Proficiency will follow only with practice and further basic knowledge.

I am indebted to the arduous labor and cooperation of the illustrator, Mr. Roger Stringham. The quality and imagination of his plates speak for themselves.

F. Richard Schneider

CONTENTS

CHAPTER 1

MUSCULOSKELETAL SYSTEM

DEFINITION

The musculoskeletal system in a strict sense pertains to muscle and skeleton, and thus bone. The musculoskeletal system is best defined, however, as a dynamic group of tissues providing structural support, allowing for voluntary motion, and giving protection to vital organs of the body. The rigidity of bones in the lower extremities makes standing possible, for without this structural support man would join "the heap" (Fig. 1-1). The contractibility of muscles in combination with the bones allows voluntary motion to take place at the joints. The osseous elements of the vertebral column and the intervertebral disks form a structural column of support for the body and also a protective canal for the spinal cord and the spinal nerves (Fig. 1-2). The histologist might refer to the musculoskeletal system as just bone and muscular tissue, while the orthopaedist defines a functional unit including tissues such as bone, cartilage, muscle, tendon, ligament, and the associated blood vessels and nerves.

DEVELOPMENT

The embryo develops rapidly from the fertilized egg and differentiates into three basic types of tissue, which then further specialize. These three tissue types are the ectoderm, the entoderm, and the mesoderm. Ectodermal tissue eventually differentiates into nerve tissue, which includes the brain, spinal cord, and peripheral nervous system. Skin is also an end-product of this tissue type. Entodermal tissue forms the gastrointestinal tract and associated structures such as the liver and gallbladder. The mesodermal tissue ultimately forms the tissue types with which orthopaedic surgery most specifically deals.

MESODERMAL TISSUE

The primitive mesodermal cells have the capacity to become a number of different cell types. They can form synovial cells that line certain joints and tendon sheaths. They are the source of the bone marrow cells that produce

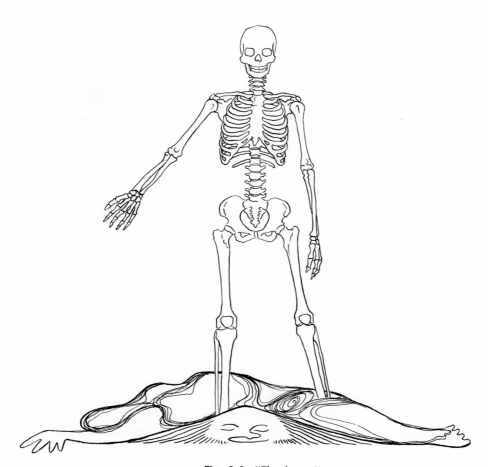

Fig. 1-1. "The heap."

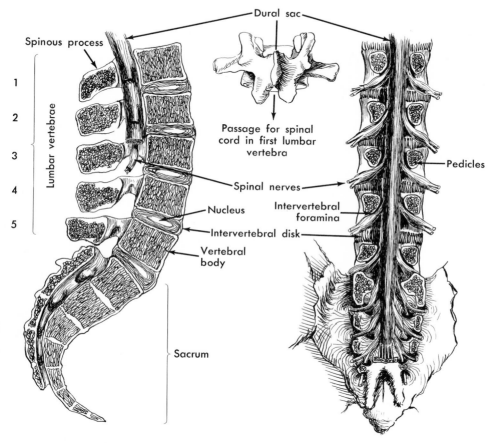

Fig. 1-2. Lumbar vertebral column provides protective canal for dural sac and spinal nerves.

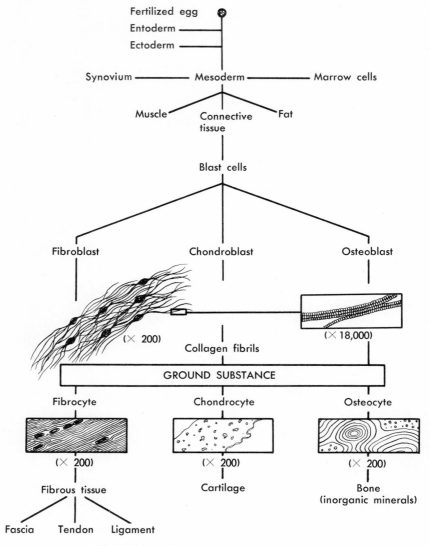

Fig. 1-3. Development of connective tissue.

the many types of blood cells in the body. The mesodermal cells can differentiate into muscle cells and fat cells as well as develop into "blast" forms for the development of connective tissue (Fig. 1-3).

Connective tissue

The connective tissues are fibrous tissue, cartilage, and bone. Although the physical properties of these tissues differ markedly, the common denominator to them all is collagen. Collagen is protein made up of chains of

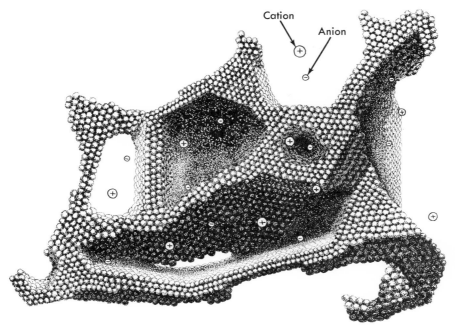

Fig. 1-4. Schematic concept of crystalline latticework.

organic molecules arranged longitudinally to form fibrils. Under the electron microscope these collagen fibrils can be seen as long strands. The connective tissues differ from one another in the types of cells and the chemical composition of ground substance in each. The relative quantities of ground substance to collagen fibrils to cells varies among the three types of connective tissue. The cell types for primitive fibrous tissue, cartilage, and bone are the fibroblast, chondroblast, and osteoblast, respectively. As each of these tissues matures, the "blast" forms alter and become fibrocytes, chondrocytes, and osteocytes. Tendon, ligament, and fascia are fibrous tissues in which the collagen fibrils are tightly arranged in parallel bundles with few fibrocytes interspersed and very little ground or intracellular substance. Cartilage has fewer collagen fibrils and a larger amount of ground substance, or chondroid, associated with more cells. The makeup of bony tissue is similar to the other two connective tissues, since osteocytes are immersed in the intracellular ground substance, namely osteoid, with collagen fibrils. Bone's peculiar physical property of hardness and rigidity is related to the deposition of inorganic crystals in the ground substance or matrix. Bone salt is made up primarily of calcium phosphate with trace amounts of sodium, magnesium, potassium chloride, and fluoride. The crystalline latticework of inorganic salts in the matrix is arranged to allow a continual exchange of these inorganic substances between the bone tissue and the re-

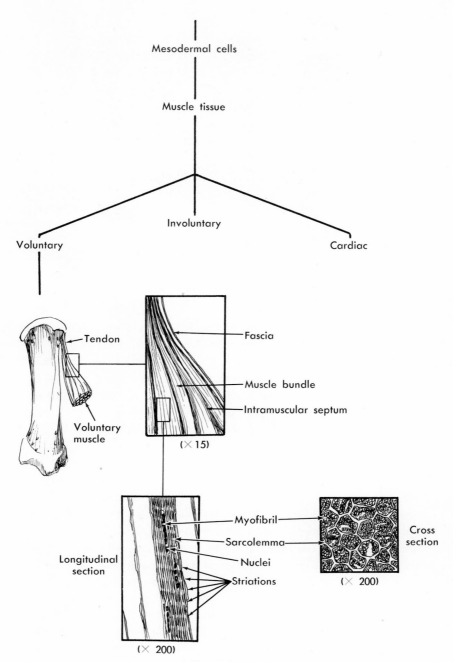

Fig. 1-5. Muscle.

maining tissues of the body (Fig. 1-4). The bony skeleton is the repository for 99% of the calcium in the body.

Muscle

Mesodermal cells may also differentiate into muscle. There are three types of muscular tissue in the human body: voluntary, striated, or skeletal; involuntary, nonstriated, or visceral; and cardiac or heart (Fig. 1-5). The orthopaedist is primarily interested in voluntary muscle. (This term is believed to be most appropriate for this type. Voluntary muscle can be brought under conscious control, in contrast to the other two, which cannot be so regulated.) The voluntary muscle fiber or cell consists of groups of parallel myofibrils in a cytoplasm or sarcoplasm surrounded by a limiting membrane, the sarcolemma. Under the microscope the parallel myofibrils have alternate light and dark areas that align with each other to give the appearance of bands or striations across the entire muscle cell. The muscle fiber is a specialized type of cell with the ability to shorten when stimulated. This quality of contractibility allows for movement, which is a fundamental function of human life. The muscle fibers are aligned in bundles to form the muscles as we see them grossly. The muscle groups are divided by fibrous tissue sheets and the intramuscular septa, and they are also ensheathed by fibrous tissue, the fascia. Muscle fibers attach directly to bone through these fibrous tissues or terminate in a tendon that then attaches to bone. In either case contractibility of muscle is transferred to bone through an inelastic tissue, and motion occurs. The initiation of voluntary muscle contraction is under cerebral control. The brain sends motor impulses via the peripheral motor nerves to the muscle, and contraction ensues.

CHAPTER 2

BONE AND BONES

GROSS APPEARANCE

The outer surface of a living bone is white and slightly tinged with pink and yellow. All bones have an outer layer of dense or compact bone known as the cortex. Within the shafts of the long bones is a medullary or marrow cavity, which contains fat cells in loose fibrous tissue called the yellow marrow. At the ends of the long bones and throughout the short bones, the cortex surrounds a honeycomb organization of osseous tissue. This cancellous bone is formed by numerous sheets or trabeculae creating multiple cavities. These spaces contain either yellow marrow or red bone marrow, where the red blood cells develop (Fig. 2-1). The trabeculae are arranged in definite

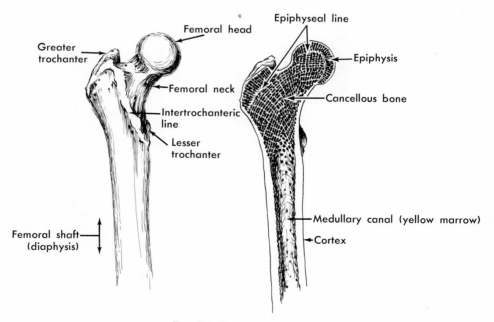

Fig. 2-1. Bone: gross appearance.

patterns to withstand the compressive and tensile stresses applied to the bone. The proximal portion of the femur has a very characteristic trabecular arrangement. Trabeculae course from the medial femoral neck into the femoral head as well as from the greater trochanteric region into the femoral head. An x-ray of the proximal femur demonstrates the crisscrossing of these groups in a manner allowing maximum strength with a minimum of bony substance.

MICROSCOPIC APPEARANCE

Microscopically, the osteocyte or bone cell is located in a lacuna or space within the calcified matrix. Each lacuna communicates with other lacunae by connecting fine channels known as canaliculi. In cortical bone the osteocytes in the lacunae are arranged concentrically around channels in bone, called haversian canals, that carry the blood supply to bone. The lacunae, osteocytes, and calcified matrix in the lamellae around the canal form a unit of bone known as the haversian system (Fig. 2-2). The lamellar pattern

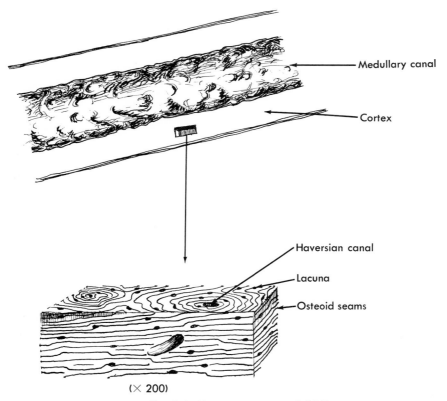

Medullary canal

Cortex

Haversian canal

Lacuna

Osteoid seams

(× 200)

Fig. 2-2. Haversian system. (×200)

of the trabeculae in cancellous bone is irregular, without orientation into haversian systems. The osteocytes in the lacunae lie in seams formed by sheets of calcified osteoid.

MORPHOLOGY

Bones may be classified into three categories by their morphology or shape. The long or tubular bones are found in the appendicular skeleton, specifically in the arms, forearms, and hands, as well as in the thighs, legs, and feet. These long bones are joined by joints, which allow for motion. The carpal and tarsal bones are illustrations of short bones and provide

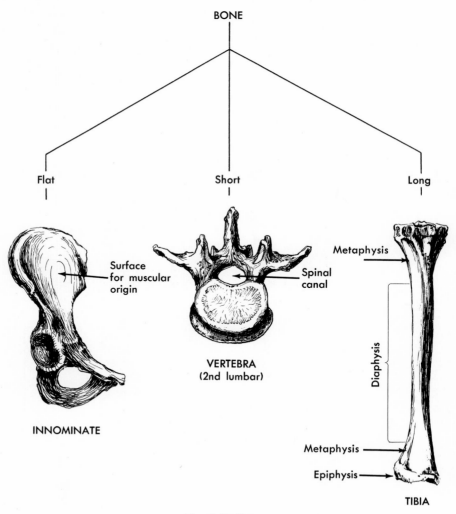

Fig. 2-3. Bone types.

special mechanical situations in both the wrist and foot for the particular function in each area. The vertebral bodies making up a portion of the axillary skeleton are also short bones. Examples of flat bones are the bones of the skull, providing protection to the brain, and the scapula and innominate bones, which have broad surfaces for the muscular attachment of the muscles controlling the upper and lower extremities, respectively (Fig. 2-3).

The bulbous end of a long bone is the epiphysis. The shaft or tubular portion of the long bone is the diaphysis. Inside the cortex of the diaphysis is the medullary canal, which in the adult is occupied by fatty yellow bone marrow. The metaphysis of a long bone is the flared portion of the bone lying between diaphysis and epiphysis.

Bony surfaces demonstrate ridges and prominences for the origin and insertion of muscles. There are also grooves to allow for the gliding of tendon over bone. The olecranon of the ulna provides the point of insertion for the triceps muscles, as does the tibial tubercle for the quadriceps muscle (Fig. 2-4). The groove behind the medial malleolus permits the posterior tibial

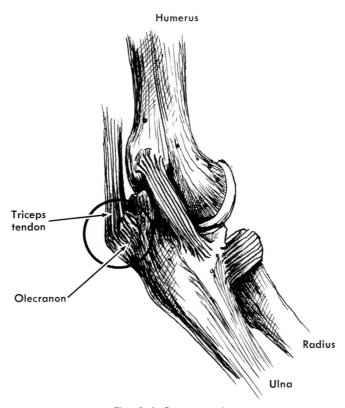

Fig. 2-4. Bony prominence.

tendon to glide on the inner side of the ankle before insertion on the tarsal navicular bone.

BONE DEVELOPMENT
Enchondral bone growth

Early in development, the human embryo develops outpouchings of tissues or limb buds that are the precursors of the arms and legs. Within the limb buds mesodermal cells congregate in the shapes of the long bones they are to form. The mesodermal cells in these models are ultimately transformed into primitive cartilaginous tissue. This primitive cartilage is made up of chondroblasts, ground substance or chondroid, and collagen fibrils. As the development of the embryo progresses, blood vessels grow into each end of the cartilaginous model at the epiphysis and also at the midportion of the diaphysis. Osteoblasts appear by differentiation at the epiphysis and diaphysis, where vascularization is taking place. These bone-forming cells produce the ground substance of bone, osteoid, as well as the collagen fibrils. The calcification of the osteoid matrix with inorganic bone salts is the final step in bone formation, known as ossification. Ossification occurs at both epiphyses and at the central or diaphyseal portion of the bone. The replacement of cartilage by bone proceeds toward each epiphysis from the midshaft until only a thin disk of cartilage remains at each end of the tubular bone (Fig. 2-5). This cartilaginous disk is the epiphyseal plate and participates in the longitudinal growth of the bone. The cartilage cells in the epiphyseal plate have the property of dividing in a longitudinal plane, thus increasing the length of the bone. Simultaneously with cartilaginous division, some cartilage is replaced by new bone, keeping the epiphyseal plate at a relatively constant width. When bone growth is complete, the cartilage cells cease dividing and the remaining epiphyseal plate is replaced by bone. The epiphyseal plate is seen on x-rays as an area of radiolucency at the end of long bones, and to the uninitiated it may be mistaken for a fracture. After the epiphyseal plate closes, this area may be recognized for a period of time as a thin line of radiodensity.

Periosteal bone development

While the mesodermal cells are forming the cartilaginous models of the long bones in the limb buds, each model becomes surrounded by an investing layer of tissue called the perichondrium. As ossification progresses, the perichondrium differentiates into periosteum, which has osteogenic capabilities or the ability to form new bone. This periosteal or appositional new bone formation increases the circumference of the long bone (Fig. 2-6). This new bone does not go through a cartilaginous stage, for periosteum is osteogenic and forms osteoid directly. After bone growth has ceased the periosteum forms a fibrous tissue layer surrounding bone except where

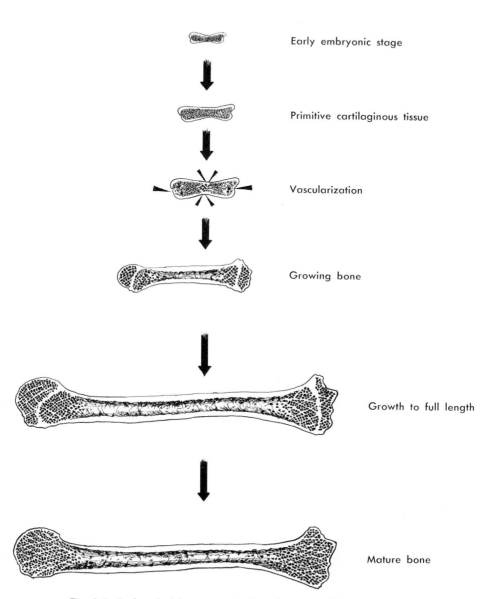

Early embryonic stage

Primitive cartilaginous tissue

Vascularization

Growing bone

Growth to full length

Mature bone

Fig. 2-5. Enchondral bone growth. Development of the long bone.

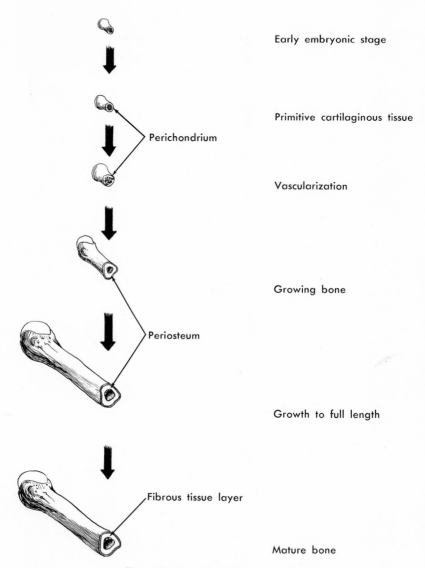

Early embryonic stage

Primitive cartilaginous tissue

Perichondrium

Vascularization

Growing bone

Periosteum

Growth to full length

Fibrous tissue layer

Mature bone

Fig. 2-6. Periosteal bone development.

the latter is covered by articular cartilage at the joints. Periosteum retains the potential to form new bone and is active and important in fracture healing.

RESPONSE OF BONE TO STRESS
Wolff's law

When bone growth is complete, the bones appear relatively static in the sense that their size and shape do not alter significantly. There is, however, a continuous process of resorption and laying down of new bone at a microscopic level in both the dense cortical layer as well as the trabecular or cancellous portion. This microscopic activity reflects forces acting on bone and in time can change the thickness of a cortical layer or the arrangement of trabeculae in cancellous bone. This remodeling of the bone in relation to stress is known as Wolff's law. Forces exerted on bone lead not only to alterations in internal structure but also to changes in external form and function. This process is dramatically demonstrated in the healing of angulated fractures in children (Fig. 2-7).

Remodeling in relation to stress

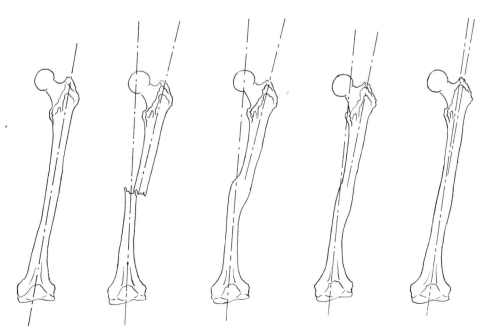

Fig. 2-7. Wolff's law.

Hypertrophy and atrophy

Bone is the densest of all tissues radiologically because of the inorganic salts or calcium phosphate content in the osteoid. If an area of bone has more stress applied to it, the tissue responds by the formation of more bone to increase strength. This functional adaptation of bone is termed hypertrophy and is seen radiologically by an increase in radiopacity of the bone secondary to the additional calcium salts. If there is a decrease in the normal stress on bone, the bone will atrophy or be absorbed, and the x-ray will be more radiolucent because of the loss of calcium salts.

BLOOD SUPPLY

The blood supply of the long bones is very rich and consists of two sets of arteries, the periosteal and the medullary or nutrient. The periosteal arteries penetrate the periosteum and enter the cortex through Volkmann's

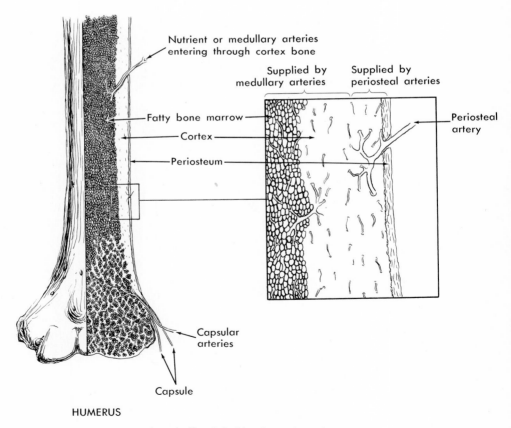

Fig. 2-8. Blood supply to bone.

canals. These arteries branch and run in the haversian systems. The periosteal blood supply supports about one-third of the nutrition of the cortical layer. The nutrient or medullary arteries pass through the cortex into the medullary canal (Fig. 2-8). These vessels supply approximately two-thirds of the cortical layer. These vessels pierce the cortex obliquely, and the holes through which they pass can often be seen on x-rays as radiolucencies. The nutrient vessels run obliquely toward the elbow joint from both the arm and forearm and away from the knee joint in both the thigh and leg, thus the rhyme: "to the elbow they go; from the knee they flee." The nutrient arteries in the intramedullary canal break up into smaller vessels that anastomose freely with each other. The blood flows through a rich capillary bed in the intramedullary canal into a venous plexus. The veins once more penetrate the cortex and connect to larger veins returning blood to the heart.

In addition to the periosteal and nutrient vessels, there are vessels that enter and leave the bone through capsular attachment at the joints. These capsular vessels penetrate and supply the cancellous bone located at the epiphyseal portion of the long bone.

CHAPTER 3

JOINTS

DEFINITION AND FUNCTION

The tissues joining two bones make up a joint. The articulations not only give the stability of one bone to another but also allow for motion between the two bones. The amount of motion and stability in any particular joint varies considerably depending on its anatomic features. The shoulder joint has marked mobility in all planes and little bony stability. This joint is held together primarily by the capsule, ligamentous reinforcements, and muscles. The intervertebral disks connecting the vertebral bodies are extremely stable joints but do not demonstrate significant motion. An additional function of the intervertebral disk is to act as a shock absorber when forces are applied vertically to the bony elements of the vertebral column. If the spinal column were a solid piece of bone without the intervertebral disks, the jolts absorbed by the feet in running or jumping would be transmitted undiminished to the skull.

Arthrology is the study and knowledge of joints. "Arthro" refers to articulations and "ology" to a branch of knowledge. Arthritis, derived from the words "arthro" and "itis," meaning inflammation, is not some magical pathologic condition. Arthritis is merely an inflamed joint resulting from a variety of causes.

JOINT TYPES
Fibrous

There are two basic types of joints. The first is a fibrous joint in which the two bones are connected by continuous intervening tissue. Although this type of joint is called "fibrous," the joining substance may not be fibrous tissue and on occasion is fibrocartilage. An example of a fibrous joint would be the intervertebral disk or the symphysis pubis joining the two pubic bones together in the midline (Fig. 3-1).

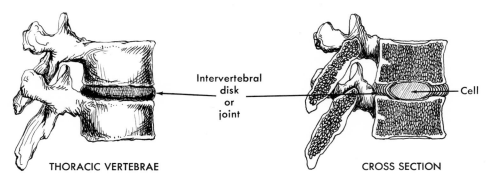

Intervertebral
disk
or
joint

Cell

THORACIC VERTEBRAE CROSS SECTION

Fig. 3-1. Fibrous joint.

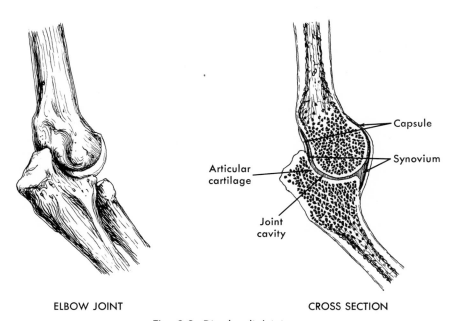

Capsule

Synovium

Articular
cartilage

Joint
cavity

ELBOW JOINT CROSS SECTION

Fig. 3-2. Diarthrodial joint.

Diarthrodial

DESCRIPTION. The diarthrodial joint is the second type of articulation and is characterized by a joint cavity between the two bone ends. Diarthrodial joints do not have continuous tissue between the bone ends. The two articulating surfaces are covered by hyaline cartilage, which is smooth, bluish-white, and resilient to pressure. The opposing surfaces are congruous and glide smoothly on each other.

The articulating bone ends are surrounded and held in apposition by a fibrous tissue capsule (Fig. 3-2). Beneath the capsule and lining the joint cavity is the synovium, which consists of a layer or two of synovial cells. The synovial cells secrete a clear viscid fluid into the joint cavity. This fluid lubricates the two opposing joint surfaces during motion and also supplies nutrition to the relatively avascular cartilaginous surfaces.

There are small amounts of synovial fluid in the normal joint. The synovium in a joint that is inflamed, however, may secrete abnormal quantities

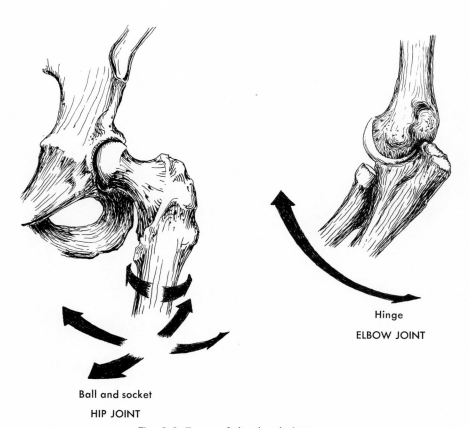

Hinge
ELBOW JOINT

Ball and socket
HIP JOINT

Fig. 3-3. Types of diarthrodial joints.

of synovial fluid into the joint cavity, producing an effusion. The normal knee joint contains approximately 2 to 3 milliliters of synovial fluid. An osteoarthritic knee joint frequently develops an effusion of 30 to 40 milliliters of clear synovial fluid. If a knee joint is injured and there is associated bleeding into the joint, the effusion is termed a "hemarthrosis."

TYPES OF DIARTHRODIAL JOINTS. The bony configuration of a diarthrodial joint often describes the type of articulation. For example, the hip joint, consisting of a socket or the acetabulum and a ball or the femoral head, is a "ball-and-socket" joint. This joint has motion in many planes, as anticipated from the bony architecture, but is partially restricted by the capsular tissues (Fig. 3-3). Certain diarthrodial joints are classified by their plane or planes of motion. The elbow joint between the distal humerus and the proximal ulna moves in only one plane and is a "hinge" joint. The knee joint is primarily a "hinge" joint moving in one plane, but it also demonstrates some rotary motion between the distal femur and the proximal tibia. Anatomically, the stability of this joint is primarily ligamentous and muscular rather than bony.

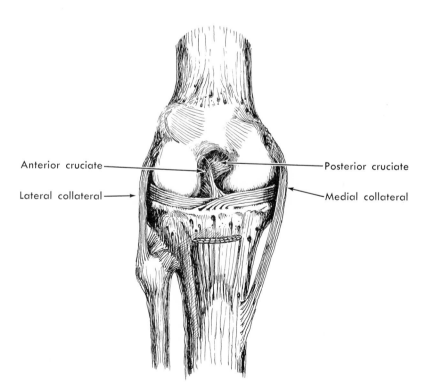

Fig. 3-4. Ligaments of knee joint. Anterior view of the flexed knee joint.

LIGAMENTS

The capsules of either the fibrous or the diarthrodial joints are reinforced in specific anatomic areas by fibrous tissue bands that create greater strength. These fibrous bands form the ligaments near a joint or joints and can be identified grossly both by anatomic dissection and at surgery.

Certain ligaments may blend in with the joint capsule, such as the medial and lateral collateral ligaments of the knee, and others may join the bone ends together within the capsule in the manner of the anterior and posterior cruciate ligaments of the same joint (Fig. 3-4).

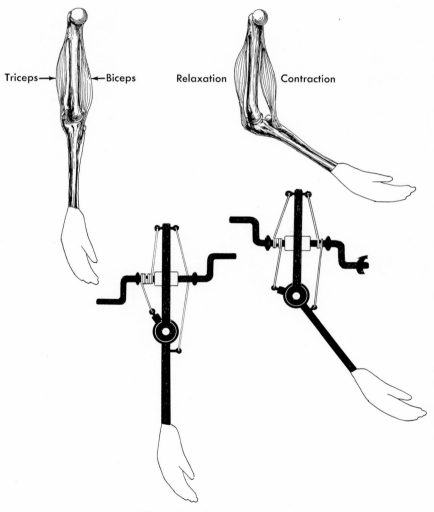

Fig. 3-5. Voluntary joint motion.

The lateral ligaments of the ankle are not closely associated with the ankle joint capsule but provide stability by their attachment from fibula to calcaneus and talus.

JOINT MOTION

Motion is produced by muscular forces acting on the lever arms of the joint. A voluntary muscle crosses the articulation originating from a fixed point on one of the bones and inserting, usually by tendon, to the other. Contraction of the muscle brings the two points closer together, causing joint motion. Voluntary motion is under the conscious control of the brain, which sends the stimulus for contraction through motor nerves to the muscle cells (Fig. 3-5).

The dynamics of joint motion are highly complex. Muscles are arranged around joints to allow not only for reciprocating motion but also for movement in various planes. The tensions or states of contractibility in these muscles must alter continuously as the joint assumes different positions. The hands playing the piano or picking a guitar demonstrate the intricate coordination required.

CHAPTER 4

FRACTURES

DEFINITION

A fracture or broken bone is a disruption in the normal continuity of that tissue. A fracture can vary from an incomplete crack through a bone to a break in which the bone is fragmented and the pieces are completely separated. Laymen will occasionally erroneously question whether there is a difference between a fractured and a broken bone. A fracture or break in bone are in fact exactly the same condition.

MECHANISM OF INJURY

Fractures are usually caused by the application of excessive stress that overcomes the normal resistance of bone. Breaks may occur from force applied along the long axis of the bone, such as a patient's fall on an outstretched upper extremity or the impact of the flexed knee against a dashboard. Torsional forces cause fracture, particularly if one end of the bone is fixed (Fig. 4-1). A ski binding that does not release the boot as the skier twists to the ground exerts considerable force on the leg with the potential hazard. Fractures are also caused by direct trauma to a part, such as the bumper of a car hitting the leg or a heavy object dropping on the hand or foot.

Bones occasionally break from forces of injury that do not seem sufficient. The possibility that a "pathologic fracture" has occurred from abnormal weakness of the bone secondary to other disease must be suspected. Treatment must be directed not only to the fracture but also to the underlying pathologic condition.

CLINICAL DIAGNOSIS
Symptoms

The possibility of fracture should be strongly suspected if the following clinical features are present: the patient relates a history of injury and complains of pain localized to an area of bone. The diagnosis is more secure if the injured part has a partial loss of function; however, the concept that

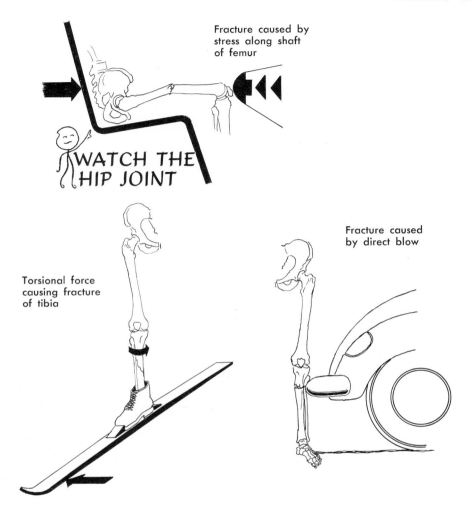

Fig. 4-1. Mechanism of injury.

there is a complete functional loss distal to fracture is erroneous. The patient with a broken forearm can move his fingers, and the patient with a fractured leg can move his ankle and toe joints. The patient who has a complete motor loss distal to a fracture of the spine or an extremity has associated damage to the nerves. The nerves are responsible for muscular activity and thus joint motion distal to the fracture. Motor function will be present, although often painful, despite the injury to the bone if the nervous elements are intact.

Signs

Inspection of the injured part reveals swelling and ecchymosis in varying amounts. Palpation demonstrates acute tenderness localized to the area of

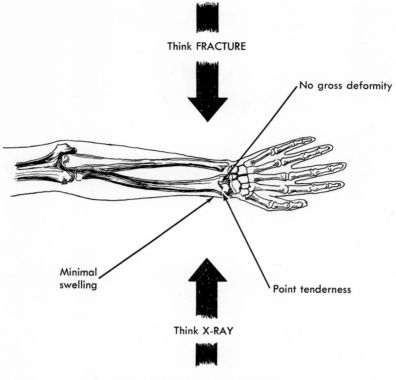

Think FRACTURE

No gross deformity

Minimal swelling

Point tenderness

Think X-RAY

Injury—Pain—Continued use of part

Fig. 4-2. Fracture diagnosis.

injury. Deformity and abnormal motion at fracture site may replace normal alignment and rigidity of bone. Abnormal motion may be demonstrated by gently moving the two ends of the fracture against each other, often creating an audible and palpable sensation known as crepitation. Angulation, abnormal motion at fracture site, and crepitation make the diagnosis of fracture quite sure, although the exact type of break cannot be determined without x-rays.

The possibility of a fracture existing without deformity, loss of function, and crepitus must be emphasized. The patient's history of injury will be the same. Examination will reveal well-localized tenderness to gentle palpation, with possibly minimal swelling in the area of injury. Function is not significantly impaired. Children often fall on their outstretched upper extremity, sustaining a torus or ripple fracture of the distal end of the radius. The evidences of fracture are sparse to nonexistent. Adequate history, thorough examination, the suspicion, and careful scrutiny of the x-ray are needed to make this diagnosis (Fig. 4-2). If the diagnosis is unrecognized and the injury not protected, an undisplaced fracture may be converted to a displaced fracture with minor additional trauma.

ASSOCIATED INJURY

When a fracture occurs, the soft tissues surrounding the bone are also injured to a greater or lesser extent. The damage to fat, muscle, and connective tissue may be sufficient to cause tissue death or necrosis. The skin can be devitalized by "degloving" or direct pressure. The soft tissue component of an injured part must not be ignored. The x-ray shows the fracture but does not indicate the severity of injury to these tissues. Considerable soft tissue swelling on the x-ray may be a clue to the magnitude of trauma involved; however, this is not specific. Careful visual inspection of the injury is the best evaluation.

The evaluation of a fracture must include particular notice of the arterial and nerve supply distal to the level of injury. The trauma causing the fracture may also damage the arteries and nerves. These structures may be contused from without or lacerated by bony fragments of the fracture.

A fracture of the femoral shaft may present with arterial insufficiency detectable by a cold pulseless foot. The uncomplicated fracture of the femur rarely causes loss of limb. The femoral fracture accompanied by an unrecognized arterial injury may require amputation.

Fractures of the distal third of the humerus are frequently associated with a radial nerve palsy. Anatomically, the nerve is bound closely to the bone in this area, allowing for mutual injury. The wrist drop that characterizes a radial nerve palsy must be recognized prior to the treatment of the fracture, for this associated injury may influence the management.

CLASSIFICATION
Closed or open

Fractures are classified as closed or open. Closed fractures do not communicate with the external environment through a break in the skin cover. For many years this type of fracture was called a "simple fracture"; however, this terminology was misleading. Closed fractures may be extremely difficult to manage and have unsatisfactory results. Open fractures, formerly designated as "compound," do communicate through the skin to the outside environment (Fig. 4-3).

OPEN: FROM WITHIN OR WITHOUT. Open fractures can result from acute angulation at the fracture site. The bone ends penetrate the soft tissues and skin from within; however, they frequently replace themselves after the forces of injury have ceased. Later examination may reveal an innocuous skin laceration even though the underlying fracture has been contaminated by bacteria. Open fractures may also be caused by penetration of the skin from without. A bullet entering the body may strike bone, causing it to

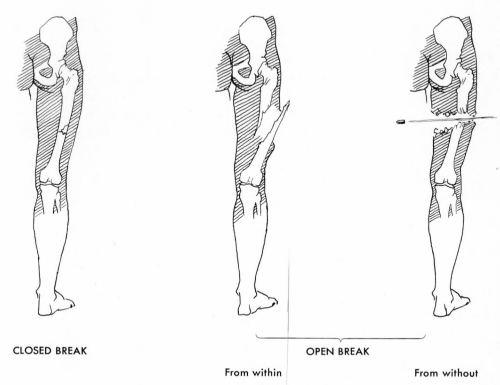

CLOSED BREAK

OPEN BREAK

From within   From without

Fig. 4-3. Closed versus open fracture.

break. Bacterial contamination is usually greater in an open fracture from without than one from within.

Infection. The external environment normally contains large numbers of bacterial organisms. These microorganisms are harmless in this location. However, if they gain access to a fracture site and multiply, a serious infection may result. Osteomyelitis or infection of bone is most difficult to eradicate. Infections in other tissues can usually be cured by surgical incision and drainage or the use of parenteral antibiotics. A resistant osteomyelitis may be uncontrollable without the total excision of the infected portion of bone. Such a radical sequestrectomy may result in marked loss of function. Serious residual disability still results from osteomyelitis despite the tremendous advances in the treatment, both by surgery and by an ever-expanding choice of antibiotics.

Descriptive terminology

Fractures are characterized by many descriptive terms. Fractures of a long bone are "proximal," "middle," or "distal," depending on the location. A fracture is "undisplaced" or "displaced," determined by the separation of

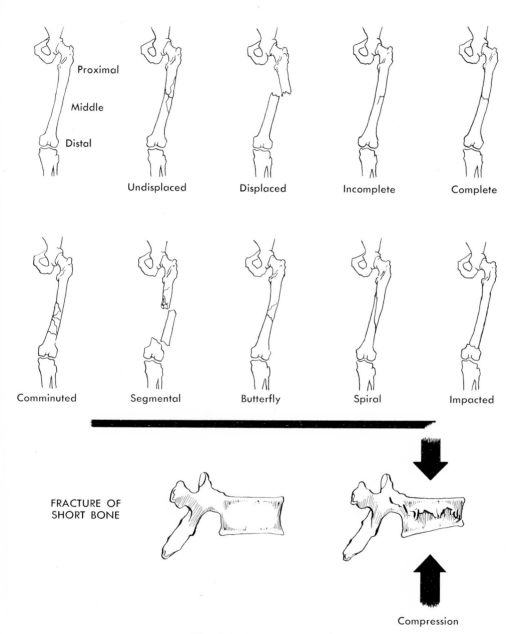

Fig. 4-4. Fracture terminology.

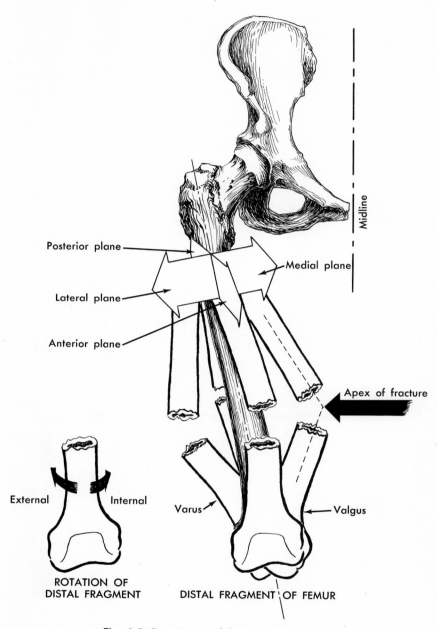

Fig. 4-5. Description of fracture deformity.

the fracture fragments. Fractures are "complete" or "incomplete" if the discontinuity of tissue does or does not go through the entire thickness of bone. A "comminuted" fracture has multiple fracture lines, thus creating more than two bony fragments. The shaft of the long bone is broken both proximally and distally in a "segmental" fracture, creating a free intervening fragment. A "segmental" piece between the main fragments is often triangular and is a "butterfly" fragment. Fracture lines may be "transverse," "oblique," or "spiral" to the long axis of a bone. A "transverse-oblique" fracture line combines both directions in one break. The two bone ends in a complete transverse fracture of a shaft lying cortex to cortex with some shortening is termed "bayonet" or "side-to-side" apposition. If the fracture fragments are driven into each other, the bone ends lock together by "impaction" (Fig. 4-4). A "compression" fracture indicates the collapse of the normal trabecular pattern in an area of cancellous or trabecular bone.

Fracture deformities

The anatomic relationship that fracture fragments have to each other is essential to the characterization of the break. Overriding or side-to-side apposition at fracture site has been mentioned. The alignment of the bony fragments in the anteroposterior, lateral and medial, and rotary planes must also be recognized. Two methods describe angulation equally well if understood and explained. The first identifies the apex of the deformity formed by the fracture, while the second method relates the distal fragment's position to the proximal (Fig. 4-5). A fracture of the forearm with the apex of angulation dorsally is a fracture with "dorsal angulation" or one with "volar angulation" of the distal fragment in relation to the proximal piece. Similarly, a fracture of the femur may present with "lateral apical angulation" or "varus (adduction) deformity" of the distal fragment in relation to the proximal. Angulation can occur anteriorly, posteriorly, medially, and laterally or the distal fragment may lie anteriorly or posteriorly, as well as into varus (adduction) or valgus (abduction) in relation to the proximal fragment. The rotational deformity at a fracture site denotes the internal or external rotation of the distal fragment to the proximal.

Children's fractures

GREENSTICK. Children's bones are less rigid than those of adults. A fracture of a long or tubular bone in a child will often break through one cortex while leaving the other intact. The injury is comparable to breaking a green twig on one side, leaving the other side intact. The "greenstick" fracture disrupts the periosteal sleeve on one cortical surface and leaves this tissue intact on the opposite side (Fig. 4-6, A).

EPIPHYSEAL INJURY. Children may fracture a bone at the epiphyseal plate prior to closure at the end of growth (Fig. 4-6, B). The displacement of a

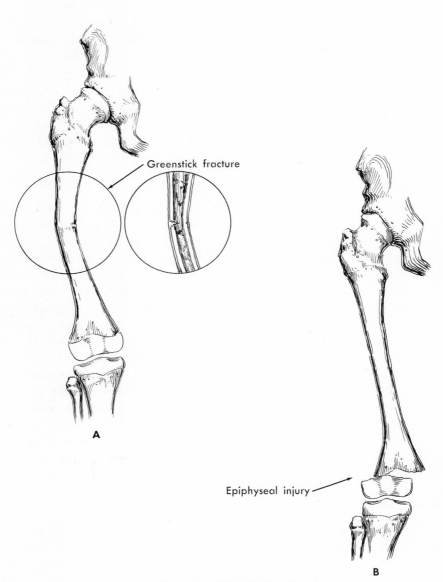

Greenstick fracture

A

Epiphyseal injury

B

Fig. 4-6. Children's fractures

bone through the epiphyseal plate causes pain and deformity indistinguish-able from a bony fracture. An x-ray is needed to differentiate the two types of injury. Separations through the growth plates are managed in accordance with the basic principles of fracture treatment. However, because of the area of injury, the possibility that growth will be altered or arrested must be considered.

CHAPTER 5

FRACTURE HEALING

Fracture healing is a unique reparative process. The fracture fragments heal or are bound together by the formation of additional or new bone at the fracture site. Most tissues in the body heal by the formation of scar tissue. If skin, muscle, liver, or brain are cut or separated, union between the two parts is by the formation of the fibrous tissue joiner, scar. New epidermal, muscle, liver, or brain cells do not develop.

SOFT TISSUE WOUND HEALING

A soft tissue injury results in lesser or greater hemorrhage. Healing is initiated by the development of a clotted hematoma, organization of the clot into granulation tissue, and maturation of the latter tissue into scar. If bones healed by fibrous tissue scar, there would be insufficient structural support provided for normal musculoskeletal function.

STAGES IN FRACTURE HEALING

A definite series of events can be observed both microscopically and radiologically as fracture healing progresses. The fact that certain steps can be identified should not be interpreted as knowledge relating to the causative factors involved. The circumstance or circumstances initiating the formation of new bone are not known. When a patient sustains a fracture of a bone, osseous union does not occur uniformly. On occasion two similar patients sustain apparently identical fractures, receive essentially the same treatment, but have varying results. One patient's fracture heals without event in the anticipated manner, while the other patient's injury fails to go on to bony union and develops a fibrous union or a pseudarthrosis. A pseudarthrosis is that type of fracture nonunion in which a "false joint" forms.

Fracture hematoma

A fracture disrupts blood vessels at the fracture site with resulting bleeding. Both the periosteal and nutrient vessels may be torn and contribute to the fracture hematoma. Within 48 to 78 hours the fracture hematoma undergoes chemical changes altering its property from a liquid substance to semisolid blood clot. The clotted hematoma is a mesh-like network of fibrin in which the cellular elements of the blood are entrapped. An abrasion of skin forms a scab in a similar manner. The surrounding of the bone fragments with the clotted hematoma is the first stage in fracture healing.

Organization of the hematoma: granulation tissue

The second development in healing is the simultaneous vascularization of the hematoma by the ingrowth of capillaries and an associated fibroblastic proliferation. The fibroblasts enter the hematoma with the capillaries. The stimulus for this vascular and fibroblastic activity is not known. The initial injury causes some tissue necrosis both by the direct trauma and by the disruption of blood supply in the area of fracture. In addition to the vascular and fibroblastic activity, phagocytic white cells move out of the vascular space into the extravascular space to absorb the products of necrosis, the fibrin network, and the other blood elements. Granulation tissue is the combination of fibroblastic activity, a rich capillary blood supply, and phagocytosis and is the precursor of scar tissue. The fibroblasts secrete the collagen fibrils and the minimal ground substance, and they subsequently differentiate into the fibrocyte. As the fibrous tissue matures, the collagen fibrils align in parallel bundles, the vascularity recedes, and the phagocytes disappear. Fracture healing may end at this stage with the bone ends joined by a fibrous and not bony union. As indicated previously, the causative factors for the continuation of bone healing are not known.

Chondroblastic and osteoblastic activity

If fracture healing progresses normally, the third event that occurs at fracture site is the appearance of chondroblasts and osteoblasts. These two connective tissue precursor cells lay down the ground substance peculiar to each and secrete the collagen fibrils in their respective matrices. Cartilage and nonossified bone consist of the proper cell types, chondrocytes or osteocytes; associated ground substance, chondroid or osteoid; and the collagen fibrils. The previously formed granulation tissue is replaced either by cartilage or nonossified bone. The relative amounts of chondroblastic and osteoblastic activity in the area of healing varies and may be related to the degree of immobility maintained at fracture site. If the fracture ends are held secure, there appears to be less cartilage formation. If bone healing continues without event, the cartilaginous elements are resorbed and replaced by bone.

Ossification: woven bone

The fourth stage of fracture healing is the deposition of inorganic bone salts in the newly formed osteoid. The inorganic bone salts form a specific crystalline latticework that is bound in a definite but as yet undetermined

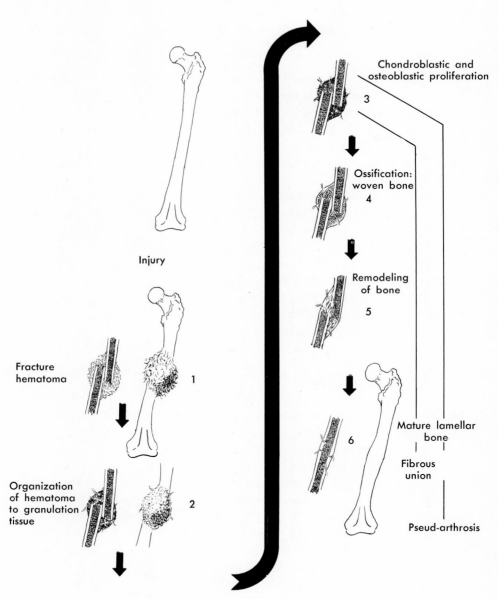

Fig. 5-1. Stages in fracture healing.

manner to the osteoid and collagen fibril. Ossification is this unique relationship of the inorganic minerals to the organic components of bone. This differs from calcification, in which the inorganic minerals are not an integral part of the tissue but are foreign and amorphous.

Microscopically, the new bone forms an irregular network without a definite trabecular pattern or haversian system. This immature ossified or "woven" bone "glues" the fractured fragments together and provides initial structural rigidity at the fracture site. This newly formed bone is the early callus seen on x-ray and appears as a homogenous density. The union of a fracture by "woven" bone is not usually sufficient to withstand unprotected stress. Bony union is incomplete, and refracture or angulation may occur when insignificant forces are applied.

Lamellar bone: remodeling

The last identifiable stage in fracture healing produces maximum structural strength. The immature bone, or "woven" bone, is replaced by mature lamellar bone oriented to this purpose. The typical lamellar pattern of cortical and cancellous bone is regained and the remodeling at a microscopic level is reflected grossly by the gradual return to the previous morphologic shape of the bone. The cortex and intramedullary canal are reconstituted. The trabecular pattern in cancellous bone develops the usual stress lines. When the fracture fragments are united by mature lamellar bone, but prior to complete remodeling, the bone is strong enough to use unprotected. At this time a fracture is clinically healed (Fig. 5-1).

After "clinical union" has occurred, the remodeling of bone continues. In children the process proceeds rapidly and in a few months or a year the previous fracture may be undetectable either by physical examination or by x-rays. Adult fractures do not have this same capacity for remodeling, and frequently the fracture site may be identified indefinitely.

The steps in fracture healing do not take place simultaneously in all areas of the repair. The hematoma formation develops uniformly with the injury, the remaining stages from vascular and fibrous proliferation to the formation of mature lamellar bone proceed at varying rates simultaneously in different locations.

FRACTURE HEALING: "SOLDERING"

The early healing of a fractured bone may be likened to the soldering process by which two metallic structures are joined together. To gain a firm and strong union requires apposition of the metals and temporary immobilization for the solder to "set" (Fig. 5-2). The same holds true for fracture healing. A fracture will unite most rapidly if there is sufficient apposition of the fracture fragments and adequate immobilization. Assuming adequate contact, fracture fragments will unite with overriding, angulation, and rotation. Actually, some shortening of the bone at the fracture site frequently accomplishes better apposition and more rapid healing. The "osteoblast" responds to the injury by the formation of new bone to form a union. With the exception of apposition, the position of the fragments is secondary.

The analogy to the soldering process is also true if the bone ends are separated or distracted. A bony bridge will be difficult to obtain and insecure when complete.

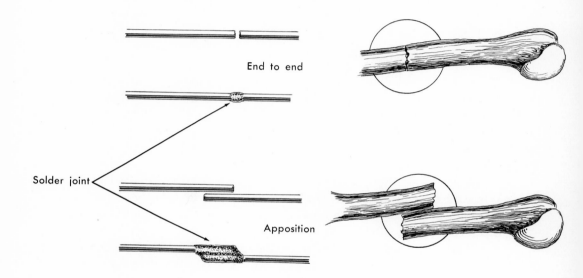

End to end

Solder joint

Apposition

Healing has no preferential alignment.

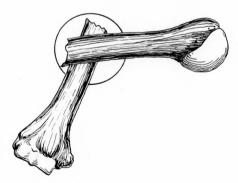

Fig. 5-2. Fracture healing—"soldering."

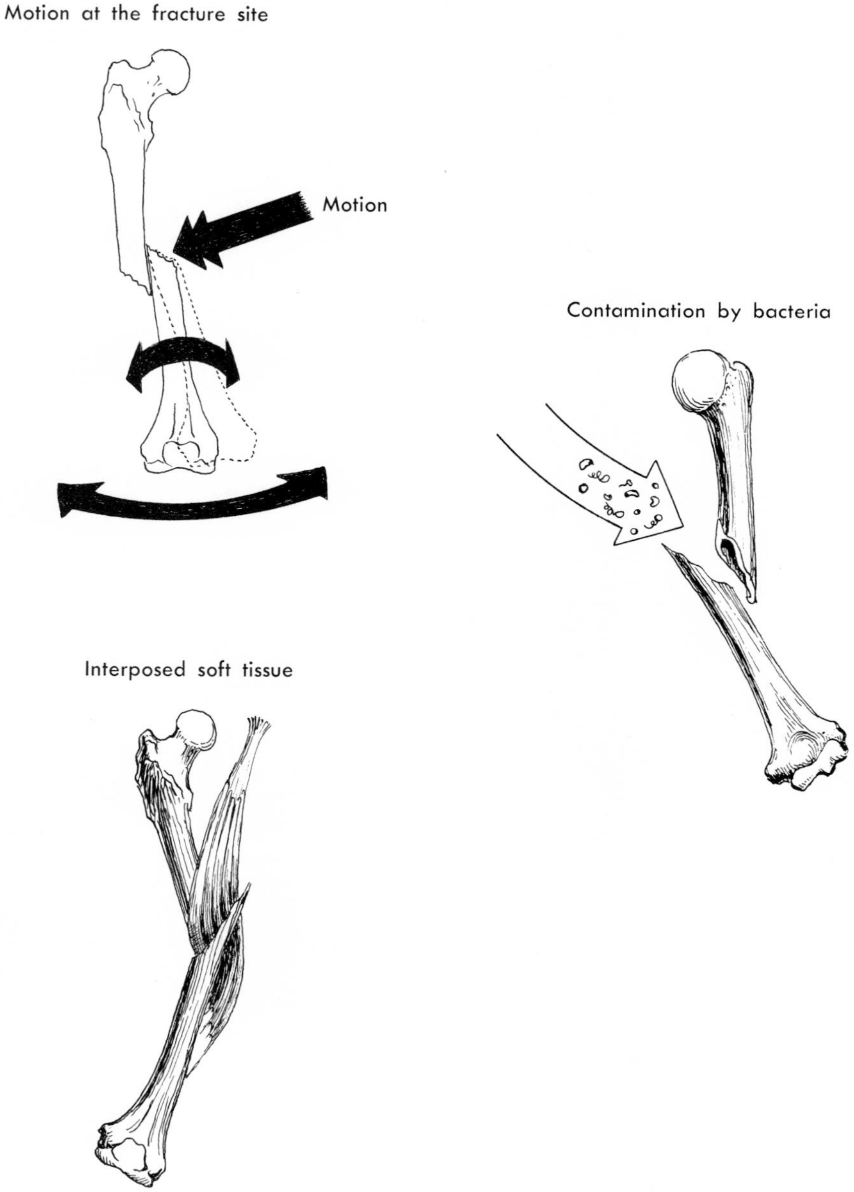

Motion at the fracture site

Motion

Contamination by bacteria

Interposed soft tissue

Fig. 5-3. Common causes for delayed union or nonunion.

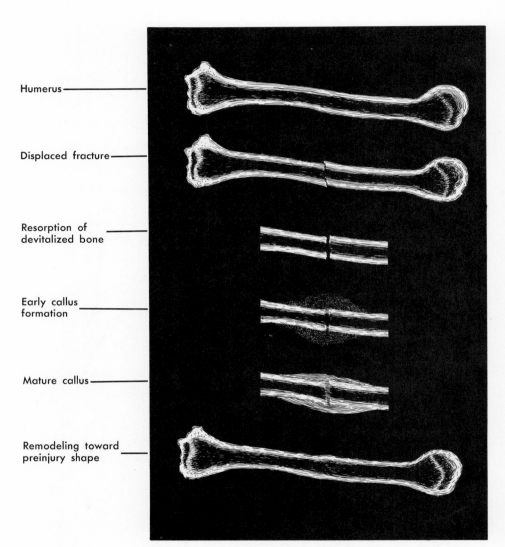

Humerus

Displaced fracture

Resorption of
devitalized bone

Early callus
formation

Mature callus

Remodeling toward
preinjury shape

Fig. 5-4. X-ray appearance of fracture healing.

DELAYED UNION AND NONUNION IN FRACTURE HEALING

Fractures that are not clinically healed in the usual length of time required for that particular bone and break are categorized as delayed unions. Nonunion denotes that the reparative process at the fracture site has ceased prior to bony union. Delayed union may proceed to complete healing without active treatment. Nonunion requires treatment to reactivate the healing process.

Certain events or conditions may delay healing or lead to the development of nonunion. If the fracture is not adequately immobilized, bony union is less likely to occur. An infected open fracture does not heal as readily as an open fracture without infection. A displaced fracture of a long bone with muscular tissue interposed between the two fracture fragments does not have the same potential for an early solid bony union as the fracture with the bone ends in good apposition (Fig. 5-3). The preceding circumstances should be avoided to enhance bone healing and prevent delayed union or nonunion.

X-RAY APPEARANCE OF FRACTURE HEALING

X-ray studies are the primary method of monitoring the fracture healing process. The determination of "clinical union" of a fracture or at what point the part may be used unprotected is based on x-ray evidence. The granulation tissue that replaces fracture hematoma causes resorption of the devitalized bone at the ends of the fracture fragments. Necrotic osteocytes, associated ground substance, collagen fibrils, and inorganic salts are removed. X-rays during this resorption phase show an apparent widening of the fracture. This gap caused by demineralization and resorption is minimal and does not impede fracture healing.

The calcification, or more correctly ossification, of the osteoid is the first radiologic evidence of healing. This early callus or "woven" bone has a homogeneous density and appears as a faint cloudiness on x-ray. Clinical union follows with the development of lamellar bone. This mature callus has a definite structural and trabecular pattern seen on x-ray and secures stable union (Fig. 5-4).

The remodeling of the healed fracture proceeds slowly over the next months and years. Serial x-ray studies demonstrate the development of a trabecular pattern related to stress, the reconstitution of cortex and intramedullary canal, and the return, at least in part, of the bone's preinjury configuration. The rapidity and completeness of these events depends to some extent on the patient's age.

CHAPTER 6

PRINCIPLES OF FRACTURE TREATMENT

THE GOAL

Fracture management strives to return an injured part to normal or the preinjury functional level. The possibility of improving on nature following an injury is unreasonable, and the concept that a bone is "stronger" after it has healed is erroneous. The injured part is rarely quite as "good as new"; however, the residual disability may be minimal, and the patient readily adapts to the deficit.

Following a severe injury to the musculoskeletal system, treatment cannot be expected to result in normal function. Just as "all the king's horses and all the king's men couldn't put Humpty Dumpty together again," physicians are unable to restore a severely injured patient without significant permanent disability (Fig. 6-1). The realization that certain injuries will result in considerable loss is important for the orthopaedic surgeon, personnel dealing with the patient, and the patient himself. Rehabilitation must conform to realistic programs and attainable achievements.

Measurements of the goal

If the goal of treatment is to return the part to as near normal as possible, the measurement of normal can conveniently be categorized to two areas.

FUNCTION. The first and most important consideration is function. This must be the first priority! The end-result in a patient with a fractured tibia and fibula must be unsupported ambulation. Treatment of fractures of the humerus, radius, and ulna must maintain and never compromise function at the hand. The upper extremity without this wondrous appendage is severely if not totally disabled. The function of injured part determines the emphasis in management.

COSMESIS. The second priority is cosmesis. The cosmetic aspects in fracture treatment must not be brushed aside as unimportant, insignificant, or frivolous. A well-shaped, straight thigh or calf should not be taken lightly. Normal appearance should only be sacrificed for functional gain. "It is not that we love cosmesis less, but rather we love function more."

PRINCIPLES

The goal of fracture treatment leads to principles in obtaining the desired result.

Do no harm: error of commission

The first principle in the treatment of any fracture is basic to all medical practice. Simply stated, it is: "Do no harm." At such time as consideration

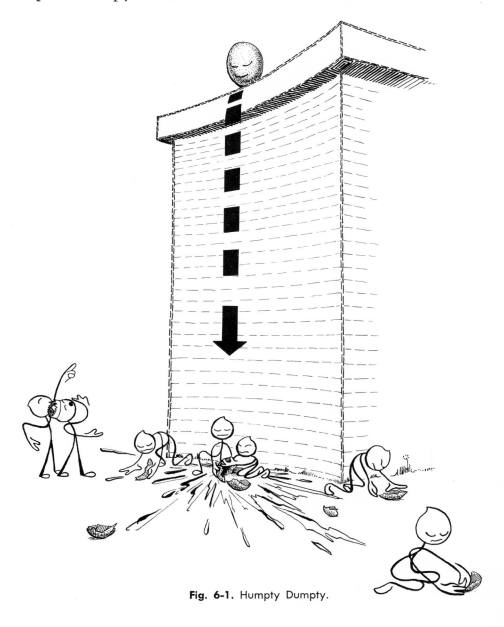

Fig. 6-1. Humpty Dumpty.

is given to "doing something," the possibility of improving the condition coexists with the possibility of causing further damage. A closed extremity fracture diagnosed clinically by deformity is not benefited by the demonstration of abnormal motion and crepitation at fracture site. This maneuver will cause the patient pain and produce further minor injury to the soft parts. Nothing has been gained. This injury should be immediately splinted to relieve discomfort and to protect the soft tissues from further damage.

This principle must permeate the entire medical management. The patient who arrives in an emergency room by stretcher must not be moved until an assessment of the consequences of such a move is made. An unconscious or comatose patient, unable to complain of pain, may have an associated undisplaced fracture of the cervical spine without spinal cord injury. The improper transfer of this patient from a stretcher might displace the fracture and cause permanent paralysis. Indeed, the patient need not be unconscious to have such a catastrophe occur, if the attending personnel do not give sufficient credence to his complaints of neck pain. Do no harm!

Take heed: error of omission

The second principle in the treatment of fractures is to take heed of the entire patient and not just the broken limb. Fractures are rarely life-threatening in themselves, and only when associated with hemorrhagic shock. Initial medical attention must be directed toward those bodily systems whose dysfunction can rapidly cause death. A multiple injury patient must be evaluated with the following considerations predominant: The patient requires an unobstructed airway and adequate ventilation to maintain life. The cardiovascular system must maintain adequate circulation to the brain, lungs, and kidneys. Hemorrhage into the abdomen from the liver or spleen will compromise this function. Deterioration of mental alertness may indicate cardiovascular failure or intercranial hemorrhage, both of which may be fatal.

The patient sent to the x-ray department with a fractured leg and other unrecognized injuries may suffer severe consequences. When such a situation is not anticipated, there is usually no resolution but only varying degrees of disaster.

STRATEGIES IN FRACTURE TREATMENT

Fracture healing is a series of events progressing to bony union. Why these steps occur in this manner and what the inciting factors are in each stage are unknown. Treatment is directed toward obtaining the ideal environment for healing. Treatment does not accelerate or make the process more efficient.

Two strategies form the basis for all methods of treatment, notwithstanding the tremendous number of fracture texts. Immobilization and reduction

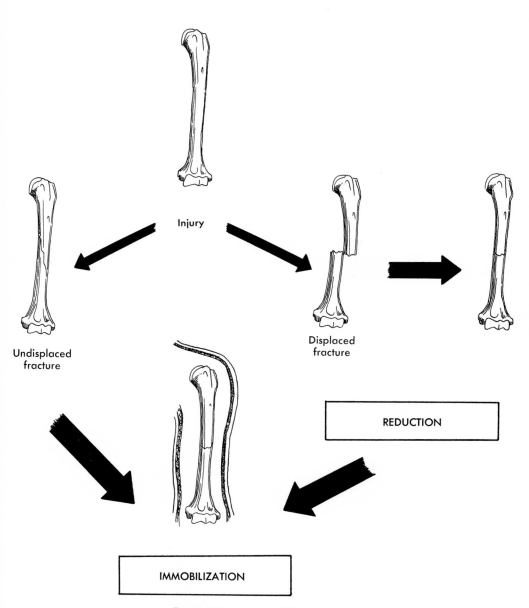

Fig. 6-2. Strategies of fracture treatment.

are the two plans of attack (Fig. 6-2). Immobilization prevents motion at the fracture site, which delays and on occasion prevents fracture healing. Reduction places the bony fragments in apposition in a functional position. Treatment by immobilization should be considered for all fractures. Certain fractures will unite without external immobilization, and these fractures are by definition stable. A stable fracture will not displace further without significant injury, is "internally" immobilized, and will proceed to bony union. Impacted fractures of the metacarpal necks, certain compression fractures of the spine, the skier's fracture of the distal fibula, and most metatarsal fractures fall into this category. Immobilization in these instances is the result of mechanical locking of the fracture fragments or from the surrounding ligamentous support. Undisplaced or slightly displaced fractures with satisfactory bone contact and alignment require no reduction. Reduction is necessary if malalignment and healing will diminish function or if inadequate apposition will delay or prevent bony union.

Immobilization

CLINICAL UNION. A healing fracture should be immobilized until "clinical union" has developed. At this point in time the fracture fragments are united by sufficient new bone to allow unprotected use of the part without the risk of late angulation or refracture. The decision that "clinical union" is present and immobilization may be discarded requires the judgment and experience of a physician (Fig. 6-3).

"Clinical union" is suggested both by symptoms and signs. The patient no longer has pain or tenderness at the fracture site. He feels the fractured area to be secure. The fracture site demonstrates asymptomatic rigidity when manually stressed, not painful motion. The most conclusive evidence of healing is the x-ray appearance of the fracture. The formation of mature callus with trabeculae obliterating the fracture is the most secure. Since an x-ray projects only one plane of the fracture, multiple views may be necessary to ensure that the fracture has healed. If just the anteroposterior (AP) and lateral views are taken, the ununited fracture may be missed. Four projections—AP, lateral, and both obliques—are required in many instances. "Clinical union" for unprotected use of the part rarely requires remodeling of the bone or reconstitution of the cortex and intramedullary canal.

DURATION. In the everyday orthopaedic practice there is an apparent cookbook approach to the healing time of any particular fracture (Fig. 6-4). Thus most finger fractures require 3 weeks, most metacarpal fractures 4 weeks, and the garden variety of Colles' fractures 6 weeks of immobilization. The analogy to the oven time for the preparation of a lamb or beef roast is obvious. This approach does not take into account the variability in fracture healing time for a specific fractured bone. A fracture that usually heals in 6 weeks, despite proper treatment, may not be "clinically united" for 8 to

10 weeks. The reasons for this delay are not known. Because unprotected and insufficiently united fractures may angulate or refracture with minimal trauma, each fracture must be assessed individually for "clinical union." The physician must decide when immobilization is no longer needed.

METHODS. Most means of fracture immobilization splint the area of injury in the desired position to a form-fitting rigid support. A plaster of Paris cast

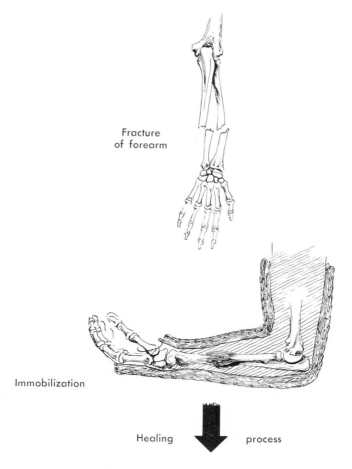

When have bone fragments united sufficiently to be used unprotected?

Fracture of forearm

Immobilization

Healing   process

When to remove? Physician decision
Lack of pain when immobilization is discarded.
Lack of tenderness to palpation at fracture site.
Asymptomatic rigidity at fracture site.
X-ray evidence of healing.

Fig. 6-3. "Clinical union."

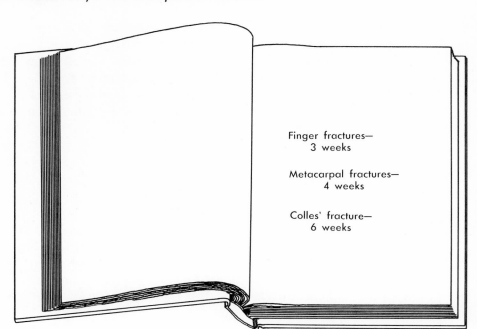

Finger fractures—
3 weeks

Metacarpal fractures—
4 weeks

Colles' fracture—
6 weeks

Fig. 6-4. Duration of immobilization.

is most commonly used for this purpose because of its accessibility, easy handling, and versatility. Metallic and plastic devices are also available and maintain immobilization in specific situations.

Immobilization by splinting is often enhanced by the simultaneous application of traction and countertraction to a particular fracture. The forces do not distract a fracture but stabilize the injury in conjunction with support or splinting. Traction is rarely applied without the associated splinting.

Adequate immobilization usually requires that "the joint above and the joint below" be included in the cast or apparatus. Absolute immobility of the fracture fragments is not obtained by any form of splinting; however, this rule promotes better fixation. A fractured distal radius and ulna maintained in a short arm cast (SAC) allows motion of the proximal fragments to be transmitted to the fracture sites. To more satisfactorily prevent motion, a long arm cast (LAC) is advised. This rationale pertains to fractures elsewhere in the body.

RESULTANT JOINT STIFFNESS. Joint function or mobility is preserved and, if decreased, improved primarily by active motion. An articulation held still for a prolonged interval becomes stiff. A joint following immobilization for an adjacent fracture is usually further disabled by additional loss of motion. A fracture must be protected until "clinical union" is secure, but not in excess of this time, for permanent joint stiffness may result. This complication is uncommon in children's fractures, and immobilization in youngsters is frequently extended beyond the normal time to be on the "safe side."

EARLY MOBILIZATION OF FRACTURES. The residual joint stiffness following immobilization is minimized by early active motion. Early joint motion may be started in certain fractures before "clinical union" has been obtained.

The impacted fracture of the neck of the humerus impales the proximal shaft into the cancellous portion of the humeral head. The fracture fragments lock with each other, creating stability. Although the fracture does not unite by new bone formation in less than 8 to 10 weeks, early motion may be advised after soft tissue healing has occurred. The fracture fragments are "immobilized" with respect to each other and bony union develops. The functional gain is better shoulder motion.

In certain fractures as healing progresses, the fragments are "soldered" together with increasing security. Although unprotected motion of adjacent joints is not advisable, gentle active motion may be indicated prior to "clinical union" to obtain an increase in motion. This decision is similar in kind to discarding of all immobilization and requires the judgment of the physician.

Reduction

The "setting" or reduction of a fracture aligns and opposes the fragments in a functional position. This is a surgical procedure whether by closed manipulation or by operative exposure of the fracture site. The indications for this surgery and the determination of the adequacy of reduction require highly skilled judgments. The tactics employed to achieve reduction are readily understood.

Closed versus open reduction

Closed reduction is the manipulation of a fracture without opening the skin by a surgical incision. This procedure is usually followed by cast immobilization. Open reduction is the alignment of a fracture by direct visualization of the bone ends. At the time of this procedure, reduction is frequently maintained by internal fixation using plates, screws, or bolts.

Closed reduction

Closed manipulation applies forces to the fracture site to obtain the optimum position of the fragments. The forces must be applied in the correct direction and in sufficient quantity to correct the deformity. The manipulation should always be controlled to prevent further injury to the soft tissues. The term "gentleness in reduction" has become popular, for it connotes the caution and care that must be exercised in moving the fracture fragments.

TACTICS. Manipulation consists of three basic maneuvers: traction and associated countertraction, angulation, and rotation. Reduction is usually accomplished by stabilizing the proximal fragment, if possible, and aligning the distal fragment to it.

The proximal fragment usually assumes a definite anatomic position depending on muscular forces acting upon it. The distal piece is deformed more often by the injury. The latter fragment is more easily controlled and placed in functional alignment with the former (Fig. 6-5).

If a traction force is applied to the distal limb of a fracture, there must

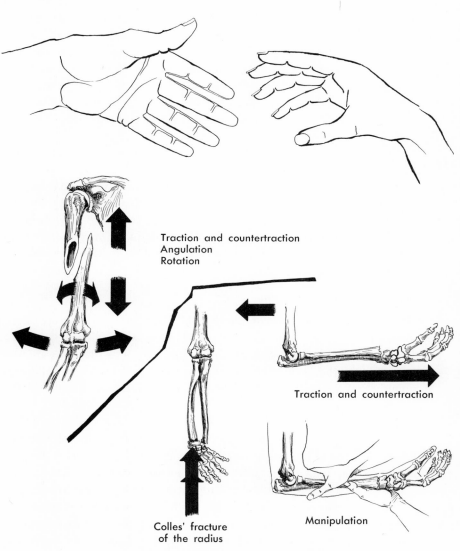

Traction and countertraction
Angulation
Rotation

Traction and countertraction

Colles' fracture
of the radius

Manipulation

Fig. 6-5. "Tactics" in closed reduction.

be opposing countertraction or the entire part will move. Traction forces should be applied gradually and steadily to overcome the muscle spasm surrounding the fracture site. Sudden stretching of the muscles increases muscular contraction and prevents ease in reduction.

PROBLEMS. Successful closed reduction of a fracture requires substantial skill to overcome the many obstacles (Fig. 6-6).

The soft tissues prevent visualization of the fracture during the manipula-

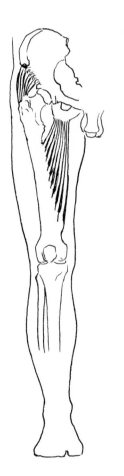
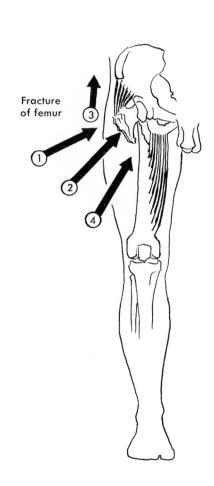

Fracture
of femur

1. Lack of visualization
2. Lack of handles
3. Muscle spasm
4. Interposition of soft tissue

Fig. 6-6. Problems in closed reduction.

tion, and proper alignment must be obtained by tactile sensation. The position following reduction is checked by x-rays; however, rarely is the procedure monitored by fluoroscopy.

The forces of reduction are not applied directly to the fracture fragments but through the soft tissues. This increases the difficulty in manipulation, particularly if the fracture is surrounded by a large muscle mass or if there is marked swelling about the fracture.

Overriding at the fracture site resulting from muscle spasm is corrected by prolonged continuous traction forces. This maneuver necessitates patience and frequently considerable strength.

The soft tissues and, most particularly, muscle may be interposed between the fracture fragments at the time of injury. Manipulation to obtain adequate bone-to-bone apposition may be comprised or occasionally prevented by this circumstance.

Ease in manipulation is hampered if both ends of the fracture cannot be controlled through the soft tissues. The proximal fragment in a femoral neck fracture lies out of reach in the acetabulum. The distal fragment of this fracture can be held; however, there is not a handle to the femoral head. Manual reduction of fractures of the vertebral bodies or pelvis is exceedingly difficult, because the fragments cannot be gripped in a satisfactory manner. The forces must be indirect and applied through joints close to the fracture.

Open reduction

Open reduction is the surgical exposure and realignment of the fracture fragments under direct visualization. This approach apparently overcomes many of the obstacles of closed reduction and affords the simultaneous opportunity to immobilize the fracture fragments with metallic devices. The benefits of this surgery must be carefully weighed against the real risks involved. The dictum "Do no harm" must be considered (Fig. 6-7).

Open reduction does not accelerate fracture healing. If closed methods fail to align and immobilize the fracture, open exposure may accomplish these goals. Open reducion is valuable to attain the ideal environment for bony union, but the fracture healing process is not altered or improved.

HAZARDS. Open reduction invariably decreases the blood supply to the bone. The dissection requires the division of small vessels surrounding the bone and also damages the periosteal vessels by periosteal elevation. Excessive interference with the blood supply may delay or prevent bony union.

Open reduction of a fracture converts a closed fracture to an open fracture, with the probability of bacterial contamination. Despite advances in aseptic technique, operative infections develop in a significant percentage of cases. A postoperative infection established in the bone at fracture site may delay or completely inhibit fracture healing. The consequence of open

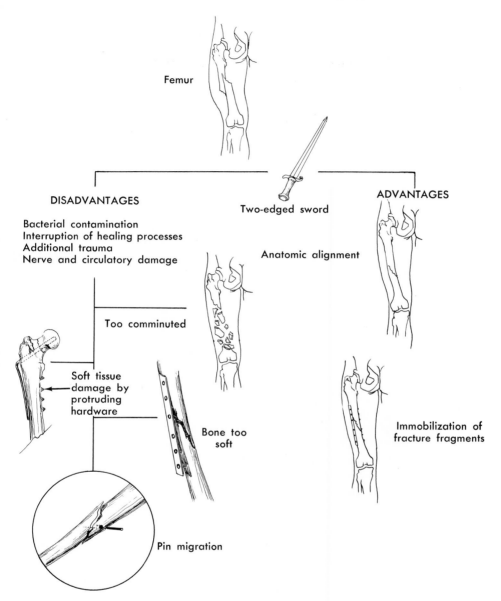

Femur

DISADVANTAGES

Bacterial contamination
Interruption of healing processes
Additional trauma
Nerve and circulatory damage

Too comminuted

Soft tissue
damage by
protruding
hardware

Two-edged sword

Anatomic alignment

Bone too
soft

Pin migration

ADVANTAGES

Immobilization of
fracture fragments

Fig. 6-7. Open reduction.

surgery may be an infected nonunion. The failure to eradicate an osteomyelitis and obtain bony union following an open reduction of a tibial fracture has resulted in a below-knee amputation.

The surgical approach to a bone is made simple or difficult depending on the proximity of vital structures. An intimately related major vessel or nerve may be inadvertently injured during surgery. This complication is not frequent, but it occurs in the best surgeons' hands and results in additional permanent disability.

Screws, plates, or rods may initially immobilize a fracture adequately. These metallic devices do not "join" with bone, eventually loosen, and fail to hold the fracture site rigidly. If bony union does not occur, continuous stress will ultimately fatigue the metals and result in breakage. This internal fixation has not been of benefit.

Extremely comminuted fractures and those in very osteoporotic bone do not lend themselves well to internal fixation. Technically, the former has too many pieces of a jigsaw puzzle to put together without excessive dissection and compromise of the blood supply. The latter fractures do not have sufficient hardness to hold the metallic devices. The immobilization obtained would be analogous to the fixation of pieces of soft butter together with a screw. If open reduction and internal fixation are attempted in these instances, the hazards far outweigh the benefits. This determination should be made before surgery.

The placement of the metallic devices may cause damage. The insertion of a screw or rod may increase the comminution of the fracture. A pin or screw protruding outside the bone may injure important vessels and nerves. Wires and pins occasionally migrate from their point of insertion to other parts of the body, causing problems.

Each decision to perform an open reduction must thoroughly consider all these possibilities.

Reduction by continuous traction

Certain fractures require continuous traction to maintain alignment and apposition of the fracture fragments. The fracture site is immobilized partially by this pull and also by local support.

A displaced pelvic fracture with one innominate bone migrating proximally can be reduced by traction and countertraction on the affected lower extremity. If the forces are released, the fracture deformity recurs. Continuous traction is necessary to maintain alignment during fracture healing.

Femoral shaft fractures angulate and shorten secondary to contraction of the large thigh muscle mass. They also require continuous traction to maintain length if closed reduction is employed.

Adequacy of reduction

Satisfactory alignment and apposition of the fracture fragments is not anatomic reduction. Although the goal is anatomic alignment, this position is not always attainable. Repeated manipulations to obtain an anatomic relationship of the fracture fragments can be harmful. Each attempted reduction increases the soft tissue damage and risks possible comminution of the fracture. A good functional result may be anticipated if fractures heal with minor angulation or shortening. Occasionally, acceptance of adequate but not perfect alignment is preferable to repetitive reduction attempts. In this instance, "the enemy of good is better" (Fig. 6-8).

A Colles' fracture is a break in the radius just proximal to the wrist joint, with impaction and dorsal angulation of the distal fragment. The ulna may or may not fracture at the ulnar styloid. The cortices of the two radial

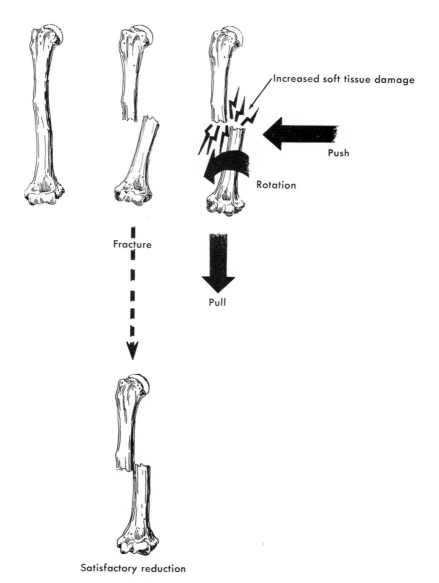

Fig. 6-8. Adequacy of reduction.

fragments are driven past each other with collapse of the normal trabecular pattern in the epiphyseal area. Inspection of a Colles' fracture demonstrates a radial and dorsal shift of the hand with respect to the forearm. The dorsal angulation presents as the "dinner fork" deformity. Anatomic reduction requires restoration of radial length. Traction forces applied to the fracture site will obtain length but also create a void in the collapsed cancellous bone. The honeycomb latticework does not regain its structured trabecular

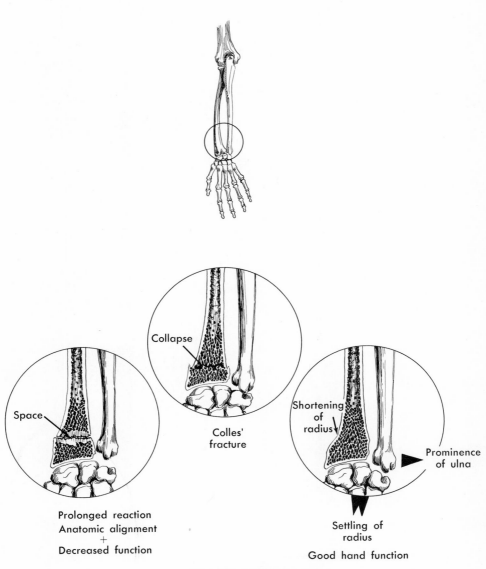

Fig. 6-9. Colles' fracture.

pattern. When the traction forces are released, the radial fracture immediately shortens without trabecular bony support. If traction is maintained during the entire healing process, the dead space will slowly reconstitute new cancellous bone. The prolonged immobilization and traction required to obtain healing in an anatomic position may severely compromise hand function. In elderly patients particularly, adequate reduction accepts some radial shortening with an associated prominence of the distal ulna to facilitate bony union and promote a useful hand (Fig. 6-9).

ANESTHESIA

The closed or open reduction of a fracture is painful and requires some form of anesthesia. The type of anesthesia will be determined by the circumstances. However, one of the following methods is usually employed.

Local infiltration of the anesthetic agent—for example, procaine or lidocaine—into the fracture hematoma frequently provides satisfactory pain relief for closed reduction. Aseptic precautions must be followed for the injection to prevent bacterial contamination and possible infection.

Injection of the anesthetic agent around nerves supplying the fracture is often adequate for both closed and open reductions. Brachial, axillary, and spinal anesthesia are in this category. These regional or nerve block techniques demand particular skills.

General anesthesia is a drug-induced, controlled comatose state in which the patient is unresponsive. Precautions must be taken to avoid aspiration of liquid.

If personnel anticipate the reduction of a patient's fracture under anesthesia, he must be placed NPO, or not receive food or water, until a definite decision is reached.

CHAPTER 7

DISLOCATIONS AND SUBLUXATIONS

NORMAL MOTION AND FUNCTION

Each diarthrodial and fibrous joint exhibits a specific and normal range of motion. The degree of mobility is determined by the anatomic configuration of the particular articulation. The continuity of connective tissues between the bone ends in a fibrous joint markedly limits mobility. The joint space of the diarthrodial joint facilitates a wider range of motion. The range of motion in the latter type of articulation is controlled by the capsule, ligaments, and the bony configuration.

Ligaments

Ligaments are fibrous bands that stabilize and restrict joint motion in certain planes by attaching bone to bone. They may reinforce an area of joint capsule, join two bone ends within a joint cavity, or provide external support to more than one joint. The medial and lateral collateral ligaments are closely related to the knee joint capsule and increase medial and lateral stability. The cruciates, which course from the intercondylar notch of the femur to the tibial spines, prevent joint distraction and control rotation. The fibular collateral ligament containing three distinct segments originates from the fibula but inserts distally to both the talus and the calcaneous. This ligament resists inversion of the ankle and subtalar joints. The garden variety of ankle sprain injures only the anterior fasciculus of this ligament, and joint stability is preserved. Complete disruption of the fibular collateral ligament permits abnormal joint motion or instability (Fig. 7-1).

Bony configuration

The bony architecture of the joint also restricts joint motion. Elbow joint extension beyond a straight line or 0 degrees is prevented by bony impingement of the olecranon process on the distal humerus. The femoral head moves freely in the acetabulum, but it is restricted when the proximal femur meets the pelvis.

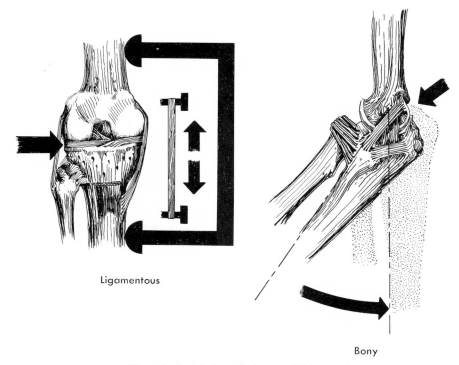

Ligamentous

Bony

Fig. 7-1. Restriction of abnormal joint motion.

DISLOCATIONS AND SUBLUXATIONS
Definition

A dislocation is the disruption of a joint in which the articulating surfaces are no longer in contact. A dislocated proximal interphalangeal joint of a finger completely displaces joint surfaces of the proximal and middle phalanges. The dislocated femoral head lies completely outside of the acetabulum.

A subluxation is an incomplete separation of the joint surfaces. The articulation remains in partial apposition, but the normal configuration of the joint is not maintained. A partial acromioclavicular separation or subluxation disrupts the acromioclavicular joint but spares the coracoclavicular ligaments. The lateral clavicular articulation is incompletely displaced cephalad from the acromion, and the articulating surfaces have partial contact (Fig. 7-2).

Dislocations and subluxations disrupt the joint capsule as well as the ligaments that stabilize that joint. A dislocated or subluxed joint has exceeded its normal range of motion, and to do so the capsule and ligaments restraining motion must be torn. The x-ray of a dislocated joint demonstrates

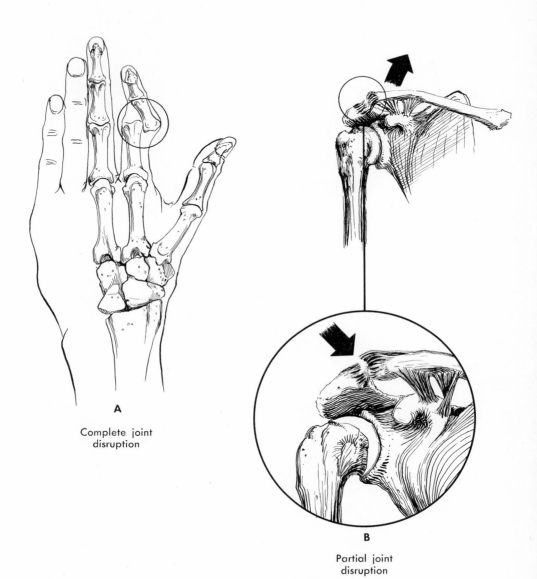

A

Complete joint
disruption

B

Partial joint
disruption

Fig. 7-2. A, Dislocation and **B,** subluxation.

only the displacement of the two articulating surfaces. The significant damage to the soft tissues is not readily evident. Proper management of these injuries requires an appreciation of the associated trauma to connective tissue, blood vessel, and nerves.

Fracture-dislocations and fracture-subluxations

Frequently a dislocation or subluxation is accompanied by a fracture of a joint surface. A posterior dislocation of a hip is often associated with a fracture of the posterior rim of the acetabulum. The loss of this buttress permits the femoral head to dislocate posteriorly from the acetabulum. This bony injury is associated with ligamentous rupture anteriorly. A common ankle fracture-dislocation includes a fracture of the distal fibula and a ruptured deltoid ligament with displacement of the talus laterally and widening of the ankle mortise. Fracture-dislocations combine fractures and ligamentous tears to create instability and displacement.

Although the clinical deformity may be typical of a specific dislocation, treatment should not be instituted without the knowledge of a related fracture. Proper management requires a complete diagnosis.

Diagnosis

The diagnosis of a dislocation or subluxation is based on the history, physical examination, and x-ray studies.

The patient describes a definite history and mechanism of injury. He complains of localized joint pain with associated loss of function. He may be aware of deformity in the injured part.

Inspection frequently reveals an obvious deformity of the joint. This abnormality is more readily appreciated if the joint is anatomically superficial and significant postinjury swelling has not occurred. Inspection of an ankle, elbow, or finger joint strongly suggests the diagnosis. Dislocations and subluxations of joints that are inaccessible to inspection may be difficult to diagnose on physical examination. Dislocations of the vertebral bodies, sacroiliac joints, and carpal bones fall into this category.

Differentiation between a fracture and a dislocation may occasionally be suspected without an x-ray. Although both injuries often present with a history of injury, localized pain, functional loss, and deformity, a fracture site shows abnormal free motion while the dislocation is partially immobile. The displaced joint surfaces and their respective bones are held securely to each other by the remaining intact ligaments. Motion at the dislocation is limited by these taut checkreins (Fig. 7-3).

Routine examination of a dislocation or subluxation must include an evaluation of the neurovascular supply distal to the injury. Any deficit should be appreciated before treatment is instituted.

DIAGNOSIS

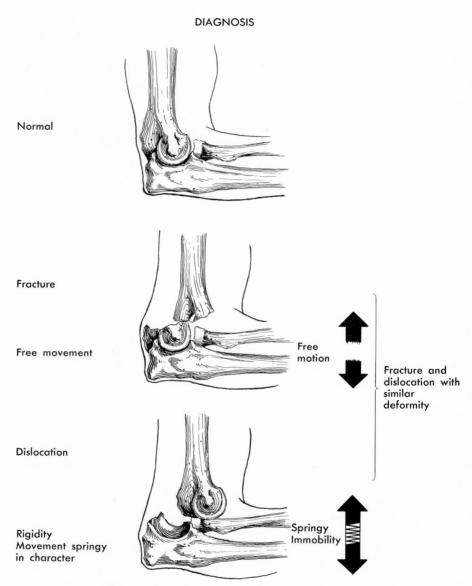

Normal

Fracture

Free movement

Free motion

Fracture and dislocation with similar deformity

Dislocation

Rigidity
Movement springy
in character

Springy
Immobility

Fig. 7-3. Clinical differentiation between dislocation and subluxation.

Pitfalls in the diagnosis

A dislocation or subluxation may pass unrecognized if joint deformity and associated springy immobility are not appreciated or if an associated injury dominates the clinical picture.

An anterior shoulder dislocation presents with obvious deformity, for the

FRACTURE ASSOCIATED WITH DISLOCATION

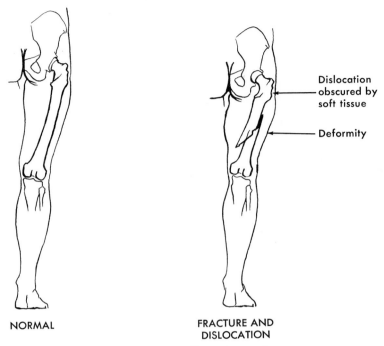

Dislocation obscured by soft tissue

Deformity

NORMAL

FRACTURE AND DISLOCATION

Fig. 7-4. Pitfalls in diagnosis.

humeral head is displaced anteriorly and inferiorly. The normal rounded configuration of the shoulder is replaced by a defect or indentation just lateral to the acromion. If the humeral head dislocates posteriorly without superior or inferior displacement, the deformity is obscured by the large deltoid muscle mass. Limited joint motion should alert the examiner to the correct diagnosis.

A dislocation accompanied by a fracture of the same bone at some distance from the joint may be unrecognized. The forces causing a femoral shaft fracture when the flexed knee is driven against a dashboard may be sufficient to also dislocate the hip. Initial attention is usually focused on the obviously deformed thigh from the fractured femur. The anatomic location of the dislocation masks deformity, and the associated fracture prevents assessment of hip joint motion. The diagnosis of the hip injury can only be made by x-ray examination. Failure to make the latter diagnosis early increases the difficulties in management and the residual functional deficit (Fig. 7-4).

Because of the inherent difficulties in arriving at such combined diagnoses, x-rays of a fractured bone should include the joint above and the joint be-

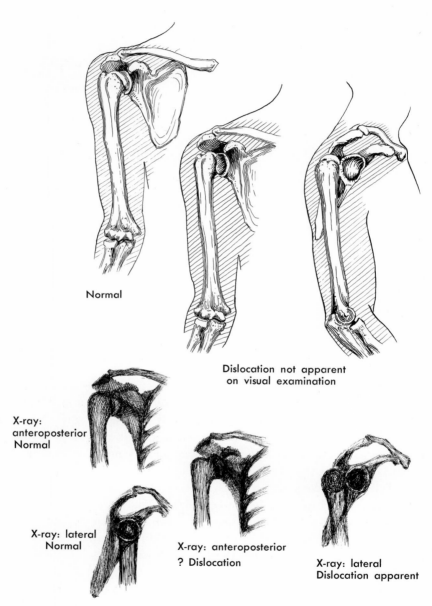

Normal

Dislocation not apparent
on visual examination

X-ray:
anteroposterior
Normal

X-ray: lateral
Normal

X-ray: anteroposterior
? Dislocation

X-ray: lateral
Dislocation apparent

Fig. 7-5. X-ray diagnosis.

low. This policy eliminates the possible unrecognized associated dislocation and its unfavorable results.

X-ray

The suspicion of a dislocation and subluxation with or without fracture is confirmed by the radiologic examination. The x-rays demonstrate either complete or partial separation of the articulating surfaces. Dislocations and subluxations are described by the anatomic relationship the distal limb has to the proximal. This displacement may be anterior, posterior, medial, lateral, or a combination of these. The ulnar joint surface lies behind the distal humerus in a posterior dislocation of the elbow. The humeral head displaces in front of the glenoid in an anterior dislocation of the shoulder.

X-rays in at least two planes are required to define a dislocation or subluxation. A single projection reflects the relationship of the joint surfaces in only one plane and may fail to demonstrate a separation in the plane at right angles. If the humeral head is dislocated posteriorly but is not displaced cephalad or caudad, a single anteroposterior x-ray projection of this joint may appear essentially normal with only subtleties to point to the diagnosis. A lateral view readily demonstrates the dislocation. A minimum of two views of any joint must be obtained (Fig. 7-5).

Spontaneously reduced subluxation or dislocation

The spontaneously reduced dislocation or subluxation is a subtle cousin of the obvious joint injuries. A traumatic force can momentarily displace the joint surfaces partially or completely. When the force ceases, the articulation surfaces spontaneously return to their normal anatomic configuration. This joint is potentially unstable and surrounded by significant soft tissue damage. Severity of injury is not evidenced by joint displacement (Fig. 7-6).

DIAGNOSIS. If a reduced dislocation or subluxation is suspected, the history should particularly emphasize the events at injury and any displacement that might have occurred.

The injured joint will be swollen and possibly ecchymotic without gross deformity. Tenderness may be localized or diffuse. Motion will be free, though limited by pain and swelling.

Controlled and limited forces applied to the joint may demonstrate abnormal motion. The stress should be sufficient to slightly sublux but not redislocate the joint. The detection of instability requires the physician's skill and experience.

Routine x-rays of the joint are normal except for soft tissue swelling. There is no residual evidence of the subluxation or dislocation.

X-rays taken during the application of controlled forces to a part are "stress films." Joint instability is determined by an abnormal relationship of the articular surfaces on the "stress" x-ray. Joint widening or shifting

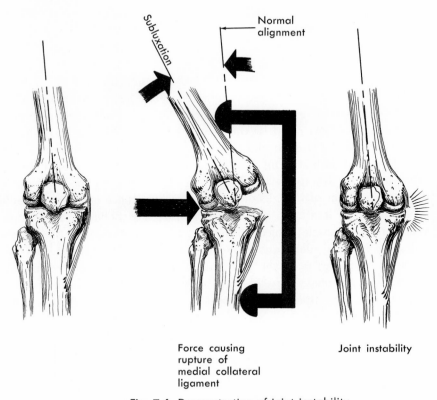

Force causing
rupture of
medial collateral
ligament

Joint instability

Fig. 7-6. Demonstration of joint instability.

beyond the normal limits confirms the diagnosis of a subluxation and possible dislocation. "Stress" studies are performed with or without anesthesia, depending on the patient's pain and cooperation. Sufficient voluntary protective muscle contraction may prevent an adequate examination, and in such a case anesthesia is required.

Complete ruptures of major joint ligaments accompany momentary dislocations or subluxations. The total disruption of the medial collateral ligament of the knee from a valgus force is associated with an initial subluxation. Physical examination and routine x-rays may suggest the diagnosis but are often not conclusive. "Stress" x-rays confirm the joint instability manifested by widening of the medial joint line.

HAZARDS. A spontaneously reduced dislocation is potentially unstable. The capsular and ligamentous supports to the joint have been disrupted, and if not protected, redislocation without additional injury may result.

A patient with a spontaneously reduced cervical spine dislocation may present with a history of injury, pain in the neck, and some restriction of neck motion but without peripheral neurologic deficit. The cervical spine x-rays will be negative. Unprotected motion of the neck may cause redislocation with impingement of the spinal cord and a resulting permanent paralysis. Such tragedies must be avoided. The diagnosis of a spontaneously reduced vertebral dislocation requires demonstration of joint instability. This consideration requires the utmost judgment and skill of the orthopaedic surgeon. The orthopaedist's assistant must be cognizant of the dangers and protect the injured part.

Treatment

The primary goal in management of joint injuries is to obtain the best possible functional result. This is best achieved by early if not immediate anatomic reduction of the dislocation or subluxation and immobilization during capsular and ligamentous healing.

Fracture healing time varies from bone to bone, depending on a number of factors. All types of fibrous connective tissue heal in approximately 4 to 6 weeks. At this time, the connective tissues are joined sufficiently by mature scar.

The initial stages in connective tissue healing parallel those of fracture healing. Thus, the hematoma progresses in an orderly fashion to granulation tissue. Here the similarity ends. The granulation tissue does not differentiate further and form additional ligamentous, fascial, or tendinous tissue; rather, it matures as fibrous tissue scar. The connective tissues are bound together by scar. In time, however, the cellular and organic components of the scar do reorganize and closely resemble the repaired type of connective tissue.

SURGICAL EMERGENCIES. Acute dislocations should be reduced as surgical emergencies. This approach most rapidly relieves severe pain and prevents further joint injury.

The articulating hyaline cartilage cells of the diarthrodial joint are nourished by the synovial fluid. A dislocation interferes with this process and may permanently damage the joint surfaces if not promptly reduced.

Joint dislocations stretch and tear surrounding soft tissues, including the vascular supply. The tension in the tissues is increased by postinjury swelling, which further compromises the circulation to bone and adjacent structures. Immediate reduction relieves tension and decreases the permanent damage from ischemia. The incidence of aseptic necrosis of the femoral head following a posterior dislocation is greater after a delayed reduction than after immediate relocation. Permanent soft tissue damage from ischemia undoubtedly occurs but is difficult to identify.

The patient with an acute dislocation should be immediately evaluated for associated severe injury and accompanying neurovascular damage. After x-rays have established the exact diagnosis, prompt treatment should be instituted.

Reduction

Reduction or relocation of a dislocation or subluxation is usually accomplished by closed manipulation. The proximal limb is stabilized as countertraction and a controlled and deliberate force applied to the distal limb. The direction of this pull should enable the joint surfaces to gently slide over each other and return to their anatomic position.

The bony configuration of the joint determines the most successful position for the application of the traction forces. Large amounts of force are not necessary if they are sustained. The muscles crossing a joint respond

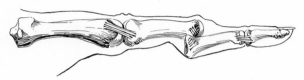

Dislocation of proximal interphalangeal
joint (PIP)

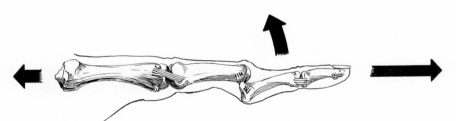

Gradual application of traction and countertraction forces
fatigues the muscles about the joint

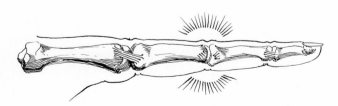

Joint surfaces realigned

Fig. 7-7. Anatomic reduction.

to the injury by spasm, thus preventing distraction of the joint surfaces. A gradual steady pull on the joint will fatigue and relax the muscles, permitting reduction. Momentary application of considerable force increases muscle spasm and hinders the manipulation (Fig. 7-7).

Reduction of the joint surfaces usually places the capsular and ligamentous tissues in satisfactory apposition for healing. The approximation of certain ligaments is improved by open suture and is recommended. A complete rupture of the medial collateral ligament of the knee with the accompanying subluxation is more secure after operative repair.

Adequacy of reduction is confirmed by x-rays. The failure to reduce an acute dislocation is an indication for open reduction of the joint. If the postmanipulation films are improved but demonstrate incongruity of the joint, soft tissue interposition must be suspected and open removal of the deterrent to reduction considered.

Anesthesia

Occasionally a satisfactory manipulation is accomplished with analgesia and gentle prolonged forces. However, frequently the severe pain and muscle spasm associated with a subluxation or dislocation prevent reduction. Anesthesia is required in these cases to permit gentle manipulation without pain and muscle spasm. Local, regional block, and general anesthesia each have specific indications primarily determined by the lactation of joint injury.

Immobilization

The reduced subluxation or dislocation with satisfactory capsular and ligamentous apposition should be immobilized in a stable position for 3 to 6 weeks. Protection is necessary following both closed and open reduction to ensure connective tissue healing. The operative suture of ligaments is insufficient without additional support.

The bony configuration of a reduced joint determines the length of immobilization. A reduced elbow joint is more stable than a shoulder joint and requires a shorter period of protection.

Splinting of the joint and gentle traction are the two most common methods used for immobilization.

The former utilizes circular or half casts and prefabricated splints. The immediate use of a circular plaster on a freshly reduced dislocation must take into account postinjury swelling and possible constriction. Sufficient padding must be applied to prevent compression. The exposed fingers and toes must be carefully monitored for circulatory embarrassment.

The use of a half cast reduces the risk of this complication but does not provide such adequate fixation. After the swelling has diminished, a change to a circular cast will provide more substantial immobilization.

Slight traction on a joint restricts free motion. The forces maintain the joint in a stable position and prevent redislocation.

Redislocation

A reduced dislocation may be unstable despite immobilization in a presumed stable position. Possible redislocation must be anticipated by serial followup x-rays (Fig. 7-8). An unrecognized redislocation may become irreducible by closed manipulation and cause severe permanent joint damage. If a redislocation is again reduced, alternate positions of immobilization or gentle traction (skin or skeletal) may be employed. If these methods are

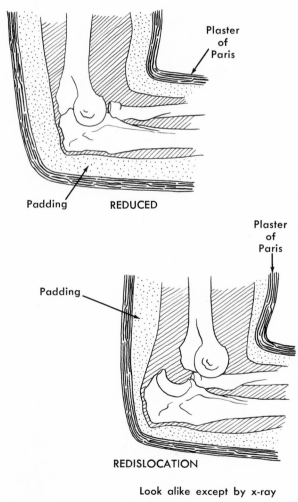

Plaster
of
Paris

Padding   REDUCED

Plaster
of
Paris

Padding

REDISLOCATION

Look alike except by x-ray

Fig. 7-8. Redislocation.

unsuccessful, reduction is often maintained by pins transfixing the joint. The internal fixation devices are removed after ligamentous healing provides stability for normal joint motion.

Rehabilitation

Joint motion is normally restricted after injury, treatment, and healing. The extent of limitation varies with the specific joint and the severity of

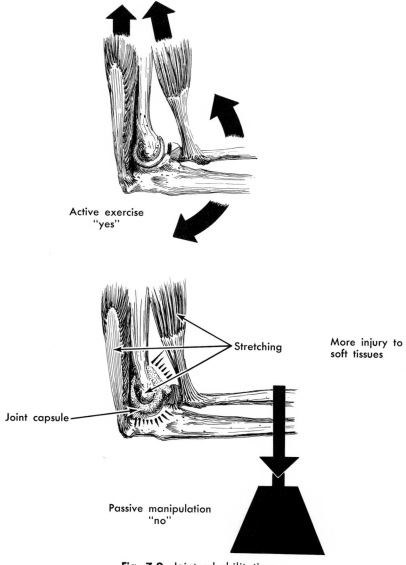

Active exercise
"yes"

Stretching

More injury to
soft tissues

Joint capsule

Passive manipulation
"no"

Fig. 7-9. Joint rehabilitation.

the trauma. A joint following dislocation will usually demonstrate less stiffening than if there were an associated articular fracture.

Fibrous scar repairs the soft tissues but also limits movement by contracture. Joint function is regained by *active* motion (Fig. 7-9).

During the healing period, the adjacent joints that are not immobilized should be actively exercised. The patient protected by a long arm cast for a reduced elbow dislocation should actively place the adjacent shoulder and fingers through a full range of motion.

After immobilization patient cooperation is essential in recognizing joint motion. Voluntary muscular contraction gradually stretches the restricting scar tissue and increases movement. Active motion of a joint may be painful, but it does not further injure the soft tissues. If restoration of motion is attempted by passive stretching, additional soft tissue injury may result, manifested by more scarring and increased stiffness. Passive manipulation of a joint to regain motion is occasionally valuable but only in expert hands.

The key to joint rehabilitation is *active* motion.

CHAPTER 8

SPRAINS, STRAINS, AND CONTUSIONS

The terms "sprain" and "strain" are sometimes incorrectly used interchangeably, leading to unfortunate confusion. A "contusion" is frequently considered to be just a "black-and-blue spot" without significant disability.

Sprains, strains, and contusions are specific injuries, and a knowledge of their pathology is necessary to render appropriate treatment.

SPRAINS

Definition

The conflicting statements that "a sprain is worse than a fracture" and "it's just a sprain and will get well" reflect a lack of understanding of the traumatic pathology involved.

A sprain is the acute incomplete tearing of capsule and ligaments from a joint injury. The forces causing a sprain may also disrupt the synovial lining with associated hemorrhage into the joint or a hemarthrosis. The involved joint is significanty injured but not rendered unstable (Fig. 8-1).

Diagnosis

When the diagnosis of a sprained joint is entertained, the possibility of a spontaneously reduced subluxation or dislocation must be considered. The correct diagnosis is reached by careful history, physical examination, and appropriate x-rays.

HISTORY. The patient complains of pain, decreased motion, and limitation of function of a joint following a sudden twisting injury. Often the immediate disability from the injury is not too severe. For example, a patient may sustain an inversion injury to his ankle during an athletic contest, suffer little immediate discomfort, and finish the game. From 2 to 3 hours later the joint becomes extremely painful and swollen and the patient is no longer able to tolerate weight on the leg.

The delayed development of severe symptoms suggests a stable joint injury. Incomplete ligamentous and capsular injury with minimal bleeding does not prevent the patient from using the part. A few hours after injury,

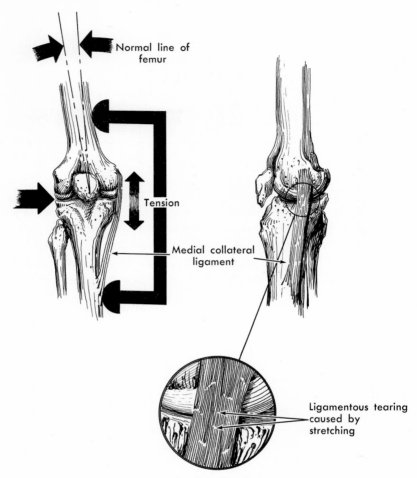

Fig. 8-1. Sprains.

however, reactive soft tissue swelling associated with a hemarthrosis may be completely disabling. This series of events occurs to a greater or lesser extent after any sprain (Fig. 8-2).

A joint that immediately loses its function after injury is more likely to be unstable. The possibility of a spontaneously reduced subluxation or dislocation with complete ligamentous rupture is greater.

The ability to immediately use a joint after injury is not sufficient to absolutely differentiate stability from instability. This determination requires evaluation of the physical findings and x-rays to include "stress" films under anesthesia when indicated.

EXAMINATION. The joint findings vary markedly, depending on the time lapse from injury. If examination is early, there may be well-localized

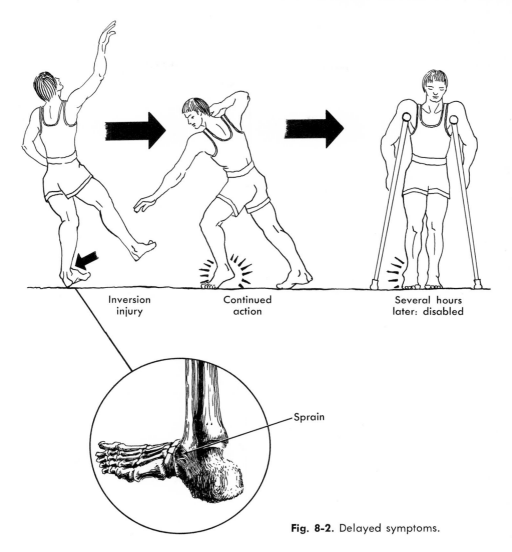

Fig. 8-2. Delayed symptoms.

tenderness to palpation but little swelling or restriction of motion. Later the tenderness will be more diffuse and associated with more swelling, ecchymosis, and limitation of joint motion.

X-RAYS. Routine x-rays will show no evidence of bone or joint injury. Soft tissue swelling may be demonstrated on the films. "Stress" x-rays are indicated if the history and examination suggest joint instability. In the case of a sprain, these studies will be negative.

Treatment

The initial management of a sprain is based on two considerations. The patient should be given maximum comfort, and swelling about the joint should be minimized. The former is accomplished by splinting of the joint in a comfortable position, the latter by a gentle compressive bandage, elevation of the part, and the immediate application of ice. Dependent hot soaks have no place in the treatment.

The most important aspect of definitive treatment is immobilization. A severe sprain weakens the ligamentous support, and so protection is necessary to prevent a complete tear from minimal trauma. The type and extent of immobilization are determined by the severity of the injury. Plaster casts should usually be applied for significant injuries. Minor injuries may be handled by an Ace bandage or soft cast to provide compression and slight support.

Connective fibrous tissue heals by mature scar in 4 to 6 weeks. Because the ligamentous injury is incomplete, immobilization for this length of time is not usually necessary and a period of 3 to 4 weeks is sufficient. Active exercise of the adjacent free joints and isometric muscular exercises in the cast promote a rapid convalescence.

After the tissues have healed, the key to rehabilitation of the sprained joint is active exercise.

Whiplash

The "whiplash" of the cervical spine is a frequently entertained diagnosis by lay people and lawyers. A "whiplash" is a sprain of the ligamentous tissues supporting the bones and many joints of the neck. There may be associated muscular damage; however, this is not severe (Fig. 8-3). The injury almost invariably is sustained by the driver or a passenger in an automobile hit from the rear by another car. The mechanism of injury is the rapid hyperextension of the cervical spine from the impact followed by acute flexion with removal of force. The term "acceleration-deceleration injury" better describes the forces involved but does not indicate the pathology.

Immediately following such an injury, the patient's symptoms are rarely severe. After a few hours, pain and stiffness develop in the front and back of the neck and progress in severity for a few days to a week. Bizarre associated symptoms often develop including headache, dizziness, visual disturbances, and nausea and are partially explained by the proximity of neurovascular structures to the injury.

Physical examination within a few minutes of injury is usually not remarkable. After an interval of time, localized tenderness and restriction of neck motion secondary to pain are in evidence. There is never any neurologic deficit.

Cervical spine x-rays show no evidence of acute bone or joint injury. There is no instability on flexion and extension views.

The cervical spine sprain should be managed by the same principles ap-

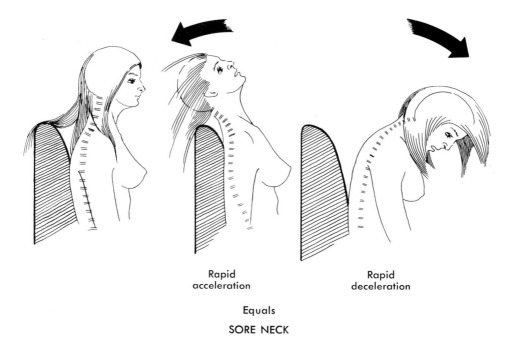

Rapid
acceleration

Rapid
deceleration

Equals

SORE NECK

Fig. 8-3. "Whiplash."

plied to other joint injury. Initial treatment is by immobilization with a cervical collar for 3 to 4 weeks, followed by active exercise. Local heat and massage may be indicated for a short period to alleviate muscle soreness, but cervical traction should play no part.

The patient's symptoms and treatment are frequently prolonged. Various socioeconomic factors including litigation may delay complete recovery. A sprained neck should not be overtreated any more than a sprained ankle.

STRAINS
Definition

A strain results from the acute or chronic use of a structure beyond the latter's functional capacity. There is not a specific injury. Most strains seen by the orthopaedic surgeon are muscular, but other tissues may be involved.

Acute muscle strain

DESCRIPTION. An acute strain tears muscle fibers from vigorous and forceful use. The contracted involved muscle is stretched acutely beyond its immediate ability to lengthen, with disruption of the tissue, hemorrhage, and associated inflammatory reaction (Fig. 8-4). The muscle damage may

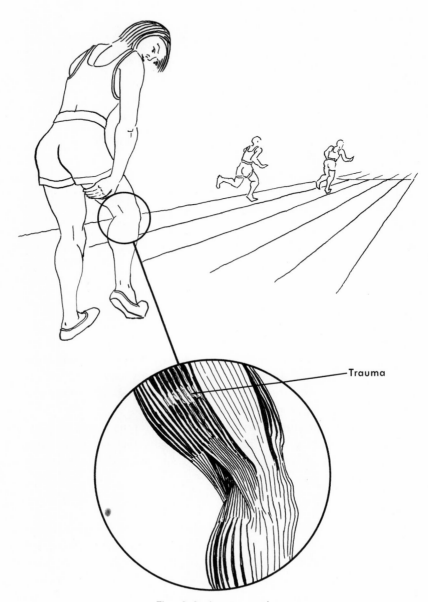

Fig. 8-4. Acute muscle strain.

be slight or, rarely, involve the complete muscle belly. Prior to vigorous exercise, progressive muscular activity "loosens" these structures and prevents strains by "warming up" to an optimal functional level.

DIAGNOSIS

History. The patient gives a history of acute, severe, disabling pain during strenuous muscular activity. A runner may "pull" a muscle in the groin, thigh, or calf during a race. After a forceful delivery a pitcher may suffer severe discomfort in the shoulder and arm. The severe pain subsides after the acute episode but is aggravated by use of the part.

Examination. The affected muscle is locally tender. Rarely will a defect be palpable even if swelling has not become pronounced. Function is limited usually by pain and not by complete rupture. Passive stretching of the involved muscle elicits discomfort. After a few days the skin becomes ecchymotic as the hemorrhage dissects to the surface.

TREATMENT. The acute muscle strain is treated by rest and, if necessary, splinting. Complete ruptures of a muscle may require open repair.

Local icepacks are recommended for the first 24 to 48 hours to decrease soft tissue swelling. After this time heat may give symptomatic relief. The damaged muscle heals in 4 to 6 weeks by mature scar tissue. During recovery muscular activity should be minimal and never sufficient to cause symptoms. The muscle may require protection with a sling, crutches, or other device.

Following healing, muscular rehabilitation by progressive exercise must be gradual. The tendency to begin vigorous activity too soon will cause a recurrence of symptoms and delay eventual recovery.

Chronic muscle strain

A chronic strain develops after repetitive use of a part beyond its accustomed performance level. The overexertion causes reversible intracellular metabolic abnormalities. The sedentary individual who takes a long hike may develop this type of strain. During the hike the person may note fatigue but only after some hours will he develop muscular aching and stiffness (Fig. 8-5).

Chronic strains have a more gradual onset, and their symptoms are less severe than acute strains. Palpation of the muscles demonstrates diffuse generalized tenderness. Function is limited by mild discomfort and stiffness. Ecchymosis and swelling are not present. Treatment of the chronic strain is expectant and symptomatic. The muscle should return to normal with rest and the passage of time. No specific immobilization is needed. Symptomatic relief is afforded by the application of local heat.

Chronic strains develop in tissues other than muscle. Joint capsule and ligament subjected to repetitive stress may not adapt to the functional load

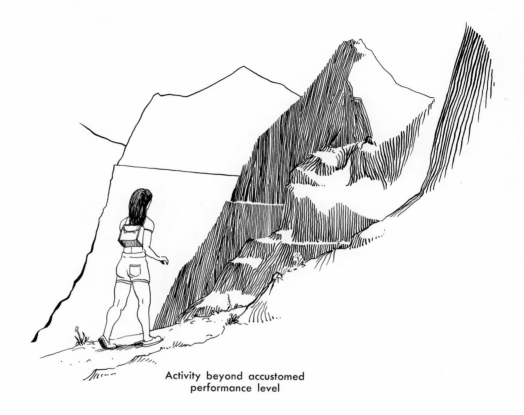

Activity beyond accustomed
performance level

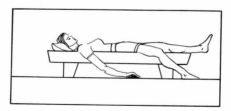

Out of commission (aching body)

Fig. 8-5. Chronic muscle strain.

and become symptomatic. The tissue tolerance is temporarily exceeded. The process is reversible if activity is decreased and the joint rested.

CONTUSION

A contusion is the result of a blow to any part of the body. The direct force may cause significant damage to skin, subcutaneous tissue, and deep soft tissues. The injury devitalizes tissues by acute compression and is associated with local hemorrhage. The latter is manifested a few days after

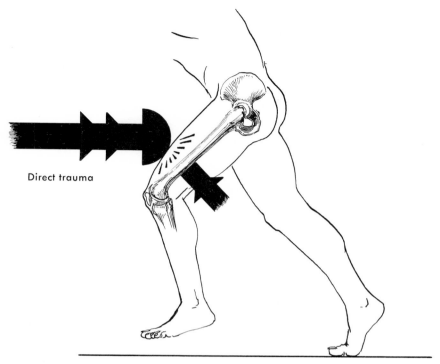

Direct trauma

Fig. 8-6. Contusion.

injury by a "black-and-blue" mark or subcutaneous ecchymosis. The extent of injury is related to the amount and direction of the external force. If the soft tissues are compressed against underlying bone, the damage is usually more severe (Fig. 8-6). Most contusions are not serious and resolve without specific treatment. The tissues are watched expectantly for any complications that may develop.

Occasionally a patient will develop marked local swelling after a blow to a muscle. The injury disrupts a major vessel in the muscle, which bleeds briskly and forms a large hematoma. The hematoma clots and is usually resorbed over a period of months. Only rarely should the hematoma be evacuated early to decrease swelling and hasten recovery. Infrequently the clotted hematoma may liquify and develop a fluid-filled space with a membranous lining or seroma. Although aspiration will temporarily collapse the sac, the fluid reaccumulates. Surgical excision of the sac may be indicated to eradicate this condition.

The physical findings of a contusion are well-localized tenderness, swelling, and subsequent ecchymosis. Adequate x-rays are necessary if the injury overlies bone to rule out the possibility of fracture.

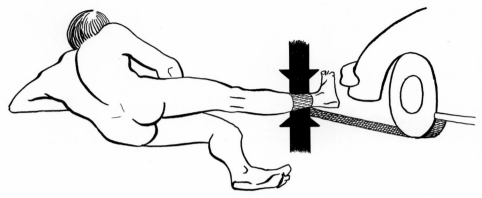

Fig. 8-7. ''Crush'' injuries.

Crush injuries

The blow causing a contusion moves the person or part away from the force. A crush injury results when the person or part is unable to move away from the force and the tissues are squeezed. A hand caught in a punch press and a leg pinned between the bumpers of two cars or run over by a car are examples of crushing injuries (Fig. 8-7). The analogy between being caught "between a rock and a hard place" is obvious.

Tissue necrosis is more extensive after a crush than after a contusion. The entire part has been compressed with possible loss of skin, muscle, and connective tissue. The reactive soft tissue swelling may be marked and embarrass the circulation and innervation.

Anticipation of the amount of soft tissue reaction to the injury is paramount to the appropriate management. An x-ray of a foot that has been run over by a car may show innocuous undisplaced fractures of the shafts of one or two metatarsals. This x-ray is the minor part of the injury. The major injury is the crush to all the soft tissues. If a cast is applied for treatment of the bone injuries without regard for soft tissue swelling, the plaster may become constrictive with the possible disastrous consequences.

Initial treatment of a crush is directed toward the resolution of swelling by elevation, mild compression, and the use of ice. The soft tissues are protected and supported by splints. Observation to determine the extent of the injury is important before definitive treatment is instituted. Definitive treatment is immobilization until the soft tissues have healed, then support and active exercises. If the crush devitalizes skin, grafting may be required to replace the loss.

Convalescence from this type of injury is slow. Pain, swelling, and joint stiffness continue for many months despite active exercise. Permanent partial disability is not uncommon.

CHAPTER 9

THINGS HEAL FASTER IN PLASTER

casts

HISTORY

Plaster of Paris mixed with water rapidly swells and forms a rigid crystalline structure. During this reaction the plaster is initially semisolid and may be molded to a desired form. The ability to shape plaster has been known for centuries; however, the Arabs are credited with its use medically for immobilization about 1000 A.D.

Plaster casts were first applied by pouring liquid plaster around a limb in an enclosed container. The hardened material conformed to the part and provided immobilization. Later semisolid plaster was spread and molded about a part during the setting process. Many people today believe this is the method of cast application.

Mathyson, a Dutch Army surgeon, developed the plaster of Paris bandage in 1852. He dusted powdered plaster into gauze bandages to act as a carrier for this material. The prepared bandages were saturated with water and applied to the part in multiple layers. This method facilitated application and resulted in a solid rigid cast.

The plaster is no longer merely dusted on the gauze, but rather various adhesives bind the material to the cloth. This prevents the loss of plaster when handling the bandages dry and controls release of the plaster during immersion.

CHEMISTRY

Plaster of Paris is derived from the naturally occurring mineral gypsum. The latter is represented by the chemical formula $CaSO_4-2H_2O$. The name "plaster of Paris" reflects the extensive deposits of gypsum found in the Paris basin in France and more specifically the Montmartre district.

Gypsum is converted into plaster of Paris by pulverization and subsequent calcination. Calcination transforms the crystalline gypsum to an amorphous state and requires high temperatures to release the water. The reaction is endothermic and is described by the following chemical equation:

$$2(CaSO_4 \cdot 2H_2O) \overset{\Delta}{\rightleftharpoons} (CaSO_4)_2 \cdot H_2O \ + \ 3H_2O \uparrow$$

$$\text{(gypsum)} \qquad\qquad \text{(plaster of Paris)} \ + \ \text{(water)}$$

The chemical reaction is reversible. When water is added to calcinated gypsum or plaster of Paris, crystalline gypsum reforms with the release of heat. This exothermic reaction explains the warmth associated with cast setting: The amount of heat given off by the cast depends on the amount of plaster used and the temperature of the immersion water.

CAST SETTING

The "setting" of a cast is the change of plaster of Paris to crystalline gypsum. The dipping of the bandages releases the plaster from the carrier fabric, primarily after application. The plaster reacts with water and forms long slender crystals that interlock with each other through the gauze layers, creating a rigid unlaminated piece of gypsum. If motion occurs during setting, the crystals will be shorter and not join as rigidly, thus weakening the completed cast.

The time interval plaster of Paris takes to form a rigid dressing after contact with water is the "setting time." The difference in setting times becomes significant as a matter of personal preference and adeptness of the operator. The cast should be applied rapidly enough to set as one unit. Various factors influence the speed of this reaction. Finely pulverized plaster combines more rapidly with water than larger granules. Warm or hot water speeds the chemical reaction. Plaster bandages thoroughly squeezed of excess water prior to application are said to set faster. If the dipping water contains residual gypsum from previous use, this will accelerate the reaction. Other substances also act as accelerators or retarders when added to the immersion water; however, chemicals usually decrease the strength of the cast.

The commercially available plaster bandages usually fall into two categories: the "fast-setting" plaster, which hardens in 5 to 8 minutes, and the "extra-fast" bandage, requiring 2 to 4 minutes.

GREEN STAGE

The plaster cast that has just set is in the "green" stage. The chemical reaction of plaster of Paris is promoted by an abundance of water; however, the water is not completely bound in the crystalline latticework. This excess water accumulates in pockets and explains the dampness and increased weight of the "green" cast. Maximum cast strength requires evaporation of the unbound water.

CAST DRYING

The cast dries by the evaporation of the excess water. The result is a mature cast containing multiple air pockets that lighten the cast and make it permeable. The skin "breathes" by these air vents through the plaster bandage.

Cast drying time depends on the amount of water to be evaporated and the thickness of the plaster. Thin casts reach maturity more rapidly than a thicker cast. Evaporation is also promoted or retarded by the surrounding environment. A "green" cast in a humid atmosphere created by a covering blanket dries slowly. The moisture evaporates more rapidly if the cast is exposed to dry, warm, circulating air. All "green" casts should be kept uncovered until dry.

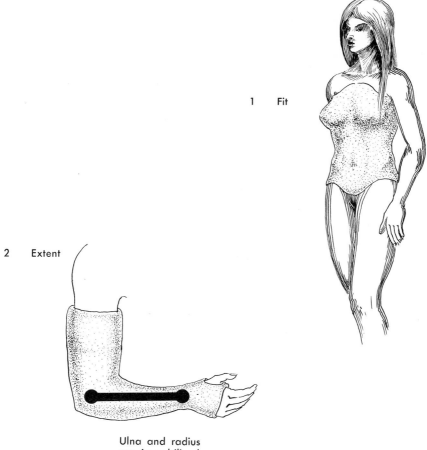

1   Fit

2   Extent

Ulna and radius
are immobilized

"joint above and joint below"

Fig. 9-1. Ideal plaster cast.

IDEAL PLASTER CAST

Plaster casts immobilize an injured portion of the body in the desired position until healing occurs. The ideal plaster fulfills this function by meeting two criteria.

The cast should have a glove-like fit and be molded precisely to the part. The underlying bony prominences and anatomic indentations should be reflected in the fashioning of the cast. Motion is possible if the plaster does not conform to these surface irregularities.

The second criterion requires the plaster to cover enough of the body to effectively immobilize the injured part. The "joint above and the joint below" should be included in the cast. A well-fitted short arm cast does not immobilize a fracture of both bones of the forearm. Elbow joint motion and forearm pronation and supination are transmitted to the fracture site through the two proximal fragments. A long arm cast is required to adequately immobilize this injury. A fracture of the tibia and fibula requires a long leg cast to control both knee and ankle joints (Fig. 9-1).

A well-fitted plaster cast of the correct length is a delight. It performs the function for which it was designed, namely, immobilization of the injured part. A poorly molded, inadequate plaster is a fraud, since it fails to do what it pretends. This is not an inherent inadequacy of plaster but rather the direct result of the clumsiness of the operator.

DANGERS AND COMPLICATIONS

Plaster casts have, by their unyielding nature, two inherent and serious dangers. To prevent complications, these must be appreciated and anticipated at the time of cast application. To realize the hazards after they have become manifest as complications, correctible or not, is neither justified nor defensible.

Pressure

SKIN. A cursory examination of the human body reveals many bony prominences from virtually the head to the toes. The malar eminences of the face, the acromion process, the olecranon, the radial styloid, the iliac crests, the head of the fibula, and the ankle malleoli are but a few that are readily palpable. These bony prominences are subcutaneous and are minimally protected by overlying soft tissues.

Cast pressure in these areas compresses the skin and subcutaneous tissues directly against the underlying bone, causing localized ischemia. Prolonged ischemia results in tissue necrosis and the development of a pressure sore. Initially the area of compression may cause pain; however, with tissue death nerves are devitalized and the patient loses his symptoms.

If a patient is recumbent in a body or spica cast, certain anatomic locations support most of the body weight. Molding of the plaster may not be sufficient to relieve this local pressure. To prevent a decubitus in the sacral area, the patient and cast must be frequently turned from side to side.

NERVE. Pressure sores are not the only sequelae of a poorly padded or ill-fitted cast. A superficial peripheral nerve may be compressed by the cast against underlying bone. Classically, the common peroneal nerve is com-

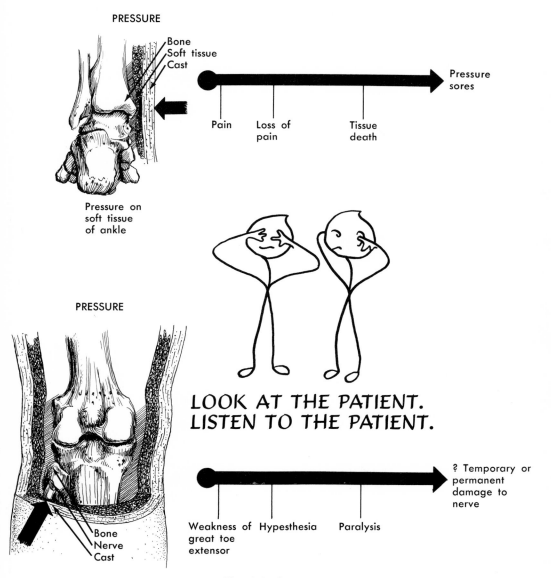

Fig. 9-2. Cast pressure.

pressed by the plaster as it swings around the neck of the fibula. This damage prevents the transmission of nerve impulses up and down and results in anesthesia and paralysis. A complete common peroneal palsy is manifested by a "foot drop" and loss of sensation on the dorsolateral aspect of the foot.

Neurologic damage may be incomplete or complete, reversible or not. As soon as a neurologic deficit is recognized, the compression on the nerves must be relieved by windowing the cast. Occasionally nerve function returns; however, this is not uniformly the case and a permanent palsy may persist.

Careful padding and molding of the plaster will prevent this serious complication. The anatomic location of the peroneal nerve must be considered during the application of all lower extremity casts (Fig. 9-2).

Constriction

Constriction of a limb is caused by circumferential rigid pressure applied to the extremity by the cast. The forces are sufficient to impede or prevent the venous and arterial circulation. When venous return is diminished and arterial flow continues, the distal extremity will become swollen and engorged with blood. If the arterial blood supply is embarrassed or stopped, the distal limb is rendered ischemic and the stage set for gangrene.

Constriction from without

Constriction may result from improper plaster application. A plaster bandage that is cinched or pulled snugly around a limb may constrict the part. The carrier fabric is unyielding, and the binding force applied by the cloth is reinforced by the plaster as it sets. The plaster must be applied without tension.

If the position of a limb is moved during cast application, the plaster already in place may be sufficiently set to constrict. This is particularly true at the elbow and knee if the joint angle is changed at an area where two parts of a cast are to be joined. The limb should not be moved until the entire cast is applied.

Constriction caused by improper plaster technique is avoidable (Fig. 9-3).

Constriction from within

The most frequent cause of constriction is swelling of the limb after cast application. An injured extremity usually swells progressively for the first 12 to 24 hours. Treatment, regardless of type, usually increases soft tissue expansion. If a circular cast is applied prior to maximum tissue reaction, venous and arterial flow may be occluded from continued swelling against the unyielding plaster. This possibility exists after circular plaster application for any injury or surgery of the extremities.

Constriction may also result from blood-soaked and clotted dressings

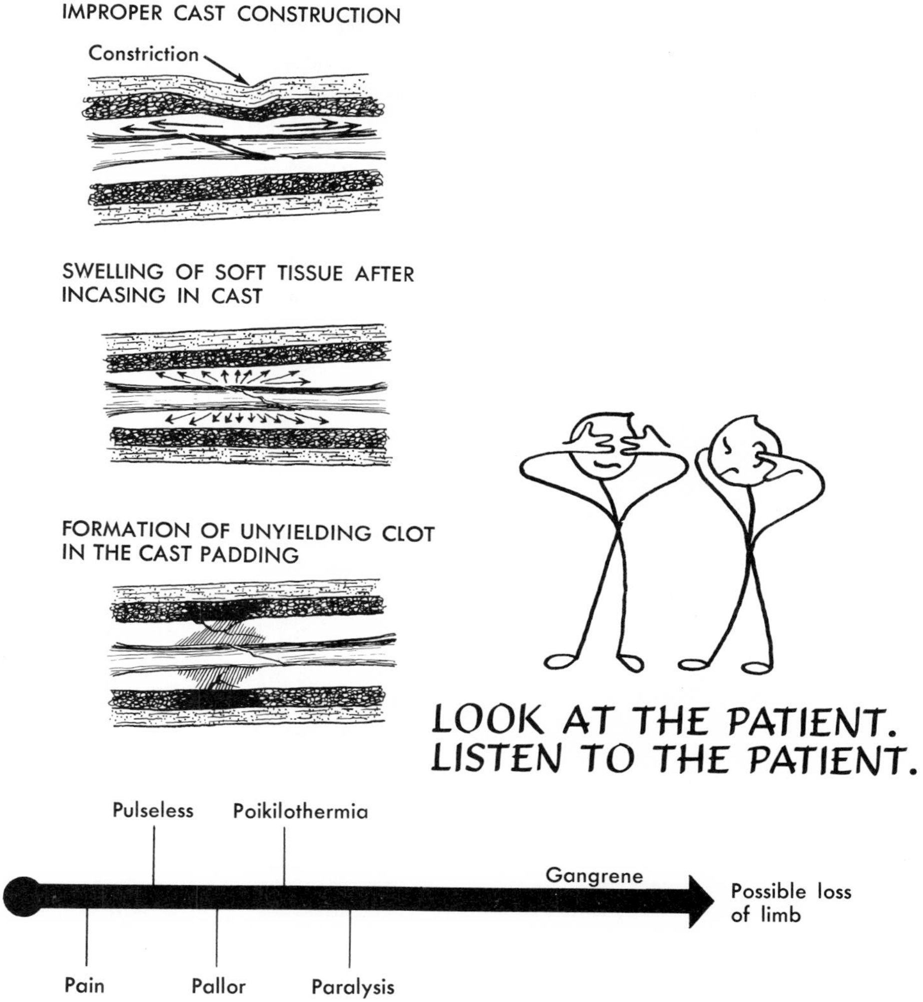

IMPROPER CAST CONSTRUCTION

Constriction

SWELLING OF SOFT TISSUE AFTER
INCASING IN CAST

FORMATION OF UNYIELDING CLOT
IN THE CAST PADDING

LOOK AT THE PATIENT.
LISTEN TO THE PATIENT.

Pulseless   Poikilothermia

Gangrene → Possible loss
of limb

Pain   Pallor   Paralysis

Fig. 9-3. Constriction.

under plaster that do not yield to the tissue swelling. These may bind the limb tightly and occlude the circulation.

These types of circulatory embarrassment might be prevented if the post-injury or postoperative cast were loose enough to permit any swelling that might develop. Unfortunately, if immobilization is required for treatment, excessive looseness of the plaster may defeat this goal. An alternative to the circular cast that avoids some of the hazards of constriction is the posterior splint or half cast, which rigidly splints only one side of the extremity. Immobilization is less adequate, but the risk of constriction is reduced. One side of the limb may swell without restriction from plaster.

Recognition of constriction

Despite thoughtful and careful technique, constriction of the extremity in plaster with distal ischemia does occur. If circulatory embarrassment is recognized early and corrected, there need be no permanent damage. Arterial blood flow to a limb may be completely interrupted for 2 to 4 hours without any residual effect. If the complication goes unnoticed, a disaster results.

The recognition of constriction begins with the suspicion. The diagnosis is confirmed by subjective and objective findings.

SYMPTOMS

Pain. Pain is the prime symptom of developing circulatory embarrassment from a cast. The patient's complaints are usually out of proportion to those anticipated after a particular injury or surgery. The pain is burning or cramping in quality and is not localized. Lack of excessive pain should not rule out constrictive phenomena, for a patient may have his symptoms masked by analgesias or demonstrate a high threshold to pain with few complaints. The evaluation of pain must be individualized.

Paresthesia. The patient may complain of numbness of the exposed fingers or toes. This sensation may be prickly, tingling, or burning in quality consistent with paresthesias.

Paralysis. The patient may or may not be aware of the inability to move the fingers or toes. The pain may be so severe as to inhibit any attempt at motion.

SIGNS

Pulseless. A cardinal finding of interrupted arterial blood flow to a limb is a loss of the peripheral pulses. The radial pulse at the wrist and the dorsalis pedis pulse on the dorsum of the foot are the usual indicators for the upper and lower extremities. The plaster cast frequently covers these sites and prevents monitoring. If vascular embarrassment is suspected, these areas should be windowed to allow for palpation of the vessels.

Circulation is also assessed by the phenomenon of capillary refill in nailbeds of the toes or fingers. Gentle pressure on the nailbed will cause blanching. On removal of the pressure the rapidity with which the nailbed returns to its normal color is an indication of the adequacy of circulation. The normal uninjured part permits comparison to determine vascular sufficiency. A pulseless limb may demonstrate adequate capillary refill in the nailbeds.

Pallor, poikilothermia, and paresthesia. The exposed fingers and toes are pale and cool with arterial insufficiency. Examining the opposite side both visually and by touch will make this evident. The digits may have decreased sensation to pinprick and light touch. Hypesthesia and anesthesia are ominous signs.

Paralysis. Motor paralysis is a late finding in the ischemic limb. The patient becomes unable to actively move the fingers or toes. Paralysis may be based on primary nerve injury; however, in this instance the other signs of vascular embarrassment are not present. Gentle passive motion, particularly extension of the fingers and toes, is exquisitely painful in the ischemic limb. A certain amount of discomfort is anticipated with such a maneuver. However, if pain is severe, vascular impairment must be considered.

Correction of constriction

The result of prolonged circulatory insufficiency may be amputation or the irreversible tissue damage of a Volkmann's ischemic contracture.

Constriction of a limb by a rigid cast or dressing must immediately be relieved by removal of the cast and the division of all padding and dressings down to skin. A cast may be bivalved and spread. However, if the padding is not divided, it may constrict. It is far better to split a cast unnecessarily than to fail to relieve constriction on a limb with circulatory difficulty. A limb has never been lost by splitting a cast and bandage and relieving the pressure.

If removal of the cast does not promptly improve the circulation, further investigation and possibly surgery may be necessary.

In summary, there is first the suspicion, then the observation and the recognition, and finally the prompt action to relieve compression.

PLASTER CAST
Setup

All of the materials required for the plaster cast should be immediately available at an arm's length. The basic supplies include padding, plaster rolls and splints, and a pail of water at the desired temperature. The types and size of padding and plaster are determined by the part to be immobilized and the preference of the operator. The padding and plaster bandages should be unwrapped and arranged for ready accessibility. There is little excuse to stop during cast application to fetch additional supplies. This time is needed to contour and mold the cast.

Any plaster residue should be rinsed from the pail prior to each cast application. This prevents the freshly dipped plaster from setting too rapidly, causing lamination and thus weakness of the cast. Operators vary in their preference of water temperature, depending on their facility in cast application. A temperature of 65° to 75° F. is recommended to promote setting in a reasonable time. Warmer water combined with the exothermic reaction from the plaster frequently causes unnecessary patient discomfort. Plaster sets too slowly in cold water and the operator's patience is tried.

In addition to the basic supplies, any materials required for a particular cast should be set out. This includes sterile dressings for wounds, special padding such as felt and sponge rubber, and devices to attach to the cast such as metallic splints, walking heels, or wooden sticks.

A cast saw, cast knife, and bandage scissors are routinely available.

The patient's position during cast application may be supine, prone, sitting, or standing, depending on the type of plaster. The apparatus used—for example, cast table, fracture table, or stool—will vary, but, regardless of which is used, each should be set up, properly covered, and stabilized.

The preparation for the cast is thorough and completed before attention is directed to the patient.

Anticipation

The patient should be advised and reassured about each step of plaster application. His cooperation is gained by recognizing and allaying his anxieties. The procedure is routine for the operator but is usually unique and undesirable for the patient.

The patient must understand the necessity of relaxing his muscles and permitting the part to be held still. If the muscles are contracted during plaster application, the cast will not fit snugly when they relax. If a patient holds his own extremity, his muscles fatigue, creating motion and often a change in position. The time spent stressing the importance of "relaxation" and "no motion" are well worth while.

Draping

The part to be immobilized must be draped with personal concern for the patient's modesty. This is possible regardless of the extent or type of the cast if given the proper consideration. The patient is correctly annoyed if he has been exposed thoughtlessly. Enough said.

Since plaster application is a messy business in most hands, the patient's clothing should be protected from spillage. He is appreciative of this consideration.

Stabilization

After the supplies are gathered and the patient properly draped, the operator is now prepared to proceed except for one most important consideration. The part to be immobilized must be placed in the required position and maintained there by an assistant or apparatus.

The operator requires both hands to apply and model a satisfactory cast. The patient should not control his own limb, for this inevitably results in motion from muscle fatigue during application. The cast will be weakened and the desired position lost. The muscles should also be relaxed for the best-fitting plaster.

The exact method of stabilizing the part is a matter of preference; however, the operator must have both hands free to apply and work the plaster.

During application, the operator must make sure that the part does not change position. This requires continuous awareness.

Padding

There are two main types of padding: cloth, represented by tubular or bias-cut stockinette, and cotton varieties, such as sheet wadding and Webril. These supplies are available in different sizes and widths to meet the specific needs. These paddings are applied directly to the skin or after the latter has been treated with a liquid adhesive such as tincture of benzoin. Skin preparation is a matter of personal preference.

Tubular stockinette is applied by unrolling a prepared length of material on the part. The cloth should extend beyond the limits anticipated for plaster application and be stretched slightly to fit snugly. The bunching of the material that occurs over the short side of a flexed joint is relieved by making a transverse cut at this level and overlapping the two edges. Tubular stockinette may be turned over and incorporated into the finished plaster, smoothing the cast's edges and preventing additional under-padding from being removed. Bias-cut stockinette is unrolled on the part with slight tension. Any wrinkles are removed by making transverse cuts and overlapping.

Cotton padding is applied in rolls with slightly more tension. The material is pulled snugly to the skin over the roll's entire surface. The roll should follow its own direction to conform to the part and not be tucked or folded. Occasionally the edge of the roll may be partially torn to round a corner; however, if the padding moves off the surface it should be torn and redirected. Many operators prefer a layer of tubular stockinette directly against the skin with additional cotton padding over it.

Regardless of the type of padding, this protection should be uniformly smooth and extend beyond the limits of the cast. Padding added after the start of plaster application is not satisfactory. Plaster applied directly on the skin is not harmful but is very difficult to remove without minor injury.

Two thicknesses of padding are usually adequate for protection and still ensure a snug plaster fit. More may be necessary, however, if significant swelling is anticipated. The part is then checked for areas such as bony prominences requiring additional protection. Increased padding of the preferred type is applied as required (Fig. 9-4).

Plaster application

DIPPING. The plaster bandage must be completely saturated to ensure that all the plaster of Paris undergoes the chemical change. A portion of the

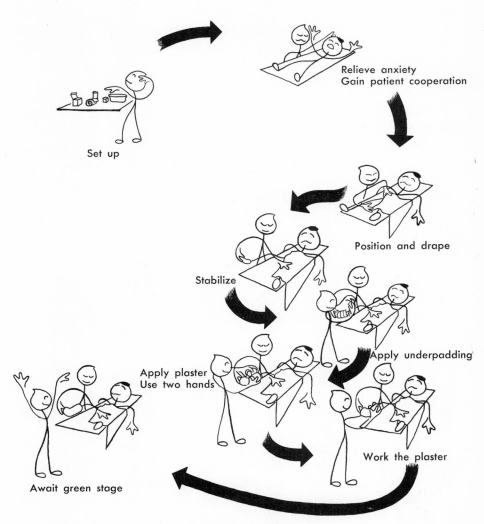

Set up

Relieve anxiety
Gain patient cooperation

Position and drape

Stabilize

Apply underpadding

Apply plaster
Use two hands

Work the plaster

Await green stage

Fig. 9-4. Steps in cast application.

excess water is immediately removed by squeezing from the bandage to facilitate application. Some plaster of Paris will be lost by this maneuver, but this should be minimized. Personal preference dictates the wetness of the bandage.

A plaster roll is saturated by placing the roll in water with one of the ends up. This position permits the free air between the layers of the bandage to rise to the surface and be replaced by water. A roll dipped transversely traps air in the bandage and prevents the water from coming into contact with the plaster.

The plaster roll is completely saturated when air bubbles stop rising to the surface. The excess water is removed by taking the bandage from the water, gripping each end to close the space between the layers, and rotating the ends in opposite directions. The vigor of this maneuver determines the wetness of the bandage. Closing the ends prior to squeezing minimizes the loss of plaster of Paris to the bucket. The end of the roll is easily identified prior to dipping and less easily so after immersion and a squeeze. The nuisance of searching for the end is prevented by making a fold or keeping a finger under the free edge while dipping.

Plaster splints are applied in units of four or five thicknesses, depending on the strength desired. Splints are saturated by holding all layers at both ends and momentarily placing them in water. The splints should not be released in the water, for they separate, tangle, and become unmanageable. The excess water is removed by holding the splints vertically out to length and then compressing them with an accordion effect on the lower hand. An alternate method is to suspend the moist splints lengthwise over the bucket by one end and use two fingers to squeeze the excess water out. This forces more plaster of Paris out of the bandage and is not recommended.

APPLICATION. Plaster rolls are used initially to surround the part and define the shape of the cast. Plaster splints are applied secondarily to reinforce specific areas in the cast.

The moistened plaster roll is placed with the outside surface on the part. The bandage is unrolled by pushing it around the part without lifting it off the surface. The plaster bandage fits smoothly if it is applied at one level to a perfect cylinder but will not if moved up or down. One edge of the bandage becomes relatively too long. Conversely, if applied to a cone, the bandage only conforms snugly without wrinkling as the bandage moves up or down and not in one position. The edge circling the lesser diameter will be loose. Plaster rolls are applied smoothly in each instance by "tucking" one edge of the plaster and thus shortening it. These tucks are created by lifting the roll off the surface without tension, catching the longer edge with a finger, and overlapping it in the shape of a V. The fold is then smoothed and the roll is replaced for further application. The tucks ensure a well-fitting, smooth cast and permit the direction of the roll. The creation of tucks eventually becomes second nature; however, practice does make perfect.

The plaster roll should never be lifted off the surface and cinched about the part. The fabric is unyielding and may cause local pressure or constriction. The slogan should be: "Push, don't pull."

The splints are laid on the part without tension. Any bunching or wrinkling is relieved by tucking or cutting a small V with scissors along an edge and overlapping the bandage. Circumferential plaster rolls hold the splints securely until the cast has set.

Five to seven layers of bandage will usually ensure a cast of adequate strength without excessive weight. The normal thickness of a cast is usually ¼ inch; however, frequently certain areas will require more plaster.

The plaster should be applied at least to the limits or slightly beyond the anticipated cast. Excess is easily trimmed, but "added on" plaster is weaker and unsatisfactory.

MOLDING. The plaster of Paris is released from the carrier fabric by water and flows in a semisolid state through the interstices of the gauze. The cast should be continuously rubbed during application to evenly spread the plaster throughout the many layers. Simultaneous molding must be carried on until the plaster has set. The flat of the hand or palm shapes the setting plaster to fit the underlying anatomy. The cast is fashioned by gentle, repetitive pressure into a surface with gradual curves. There should be no acute indentations resulting from the molding. Plaster application is a two-handed job. Both the operator's hands must be free to satisfactorily perform the task.

Although plaster of Paris forms stronger gypsum in the absence of any motion, molding only minimally decreases strength and markedly enhances the fit of the cast.

The temptation to stop working the plaster before it has completely set must be resisted. The molding must continue until the cast is rigid or the fit will not hold.

Prematurely moving the part to be immobilized may crack and weaken the plaster. Better to hold steady another 2 or 3 minutes than go back and reinforce an area. Also, the incompletely set cast indents easily if placed on a firm surface, creating a potential pressure area. This circumstance requires immediate correction, which is time consuming.

Cast trimming

Excess plaster is trimmed in the early "green stage" with a sharp scalpel and steady hand. The scalpel must be under complete control at all times to prevent inadvertent skin cuts. The blade is not pushed down into the cast but the plaster edge pulled up against the cutting edge. If the cast becomes too hard to cut easily with a knife, safety dictates the use of the cast saw.

Aftercare

Plaster on the skin is removed with a moist cloth. The "green" cast is protected from stress and supported as necessary with pillows. The plaster is kept uncovered to promote cast drying. The patient is instructed in the danger signals and advised how to care for the cast. The mess created by the application of a cast is the operator's responsibility. The supplies and equipment are cleaned, replaced, and readied for further use. Any plaster is removed from the tables and floors. The room is left at least as clean as at the onset. The man who considers these tasks beneath him should not lift a single roll of plaster.

PATIENT INSTRUCTIONS
Know danger signs

PAIN. The patient must immediately report to the physician any increased discomfort after cast application. This is true regardless of the type and location of the pain. Immediately after cast application, the patient may be concerned by the heat of the plaster. In this instance, he may be reassured that this is normal and will pass in 10 to 15 minutes.

SWELLING. Mild swelling of the exposed fingers and toes from a cast is not unusual and should be anticipated if the limb is dependent. This swelling may be reduced by elevation of the part above the level of the heart, increasing venous and lymphatic return.

Moderate swelling associated with pain and discoloration should be promptly evaluated by the physician.

MISCELLANEOUS. Any untoward medical events should also be reported to and evaluated by the physician. Nausea, vomiting, chills, fever, or a rash may all reflect a complication under the plaster.

Advise the patient

KEEP UNCOVERED. The "green" cast should be left exposed to air until mature. The drying time varies with the thickness of the plaster but is usually 24 to 48 hours.

PROTECT. A cast does not reach maximum strength until completely dry and should be protected. Upper extremity casts are placed in slings until maturity is reached. Lower extremity casts, weight bearing or not, are initially protected by crutches. The patient should be instructed not to bear weight on a walking cast for 24 to 48 hours after application.

KEEP CLEAN. The cast should be kept clean, for this prevents cast breakdown and somewhat restricts the patient from undesirable activities. The soiled cast cannot be cleaned but only covered with additional plaster or materials such as shoe polish to give the appearance of cleanliness.

Many patients enjoy decorating their casts, and there is no objection to this with one admonition. The plaster is porous and permits the evaporation of moisture from the skin. If the cast is sealed with an air-impervious material, evaporation is impaired and the skin may macerate.

AVOID MOISTURE. The cast must be kept dry. Water causes the mature plaster to crumble and become soft. The gypsum is washed out and only the gauze bandage remains. The immobilization of a cast is no longer effective. The patient in an extremity cast may take a shower or bath. The plaster is covered by a watertight plastic bag drawn close to the skin proximally by an elastic band. Commercial items are available specifically for this use.

"DO NOT"

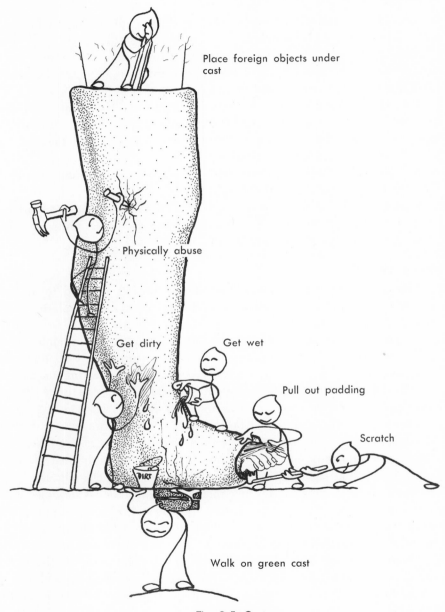

Place foreign objects under cast

Physically abuse

Get dirty

Get wet

Pull out padding

Scratch

Walk on green cast

Fig. 9-5. Cast care.

DON'T SCRATCH. Many patients develop a tremendous desire to scratch an itch beneath a plaster. Manipulating devices such as a coat hanger, back scratcher, or pencil beneath a plaster is prohibited. The relief afforded is temporary and discomfort invariably returns with increased vigor. The attempt to relieve the irritation wrinkles, wads, and bunches the smooth padded surface and may cause pressure areas. The "scratcher" also may be "lost" during the effort (Fig. 9-5).

INSERT NO FOREIGN OBJECTS. No foreign objects should be introduced under the cast. If this occurs, the physician should be notified immediately. A rigid foreign body beneath a snugly molded cast must cause localized pressure on the skin with the possibility of a pressure sore. Toothbrushes, coins, good luck charms, and many other objects have been found under casts and on occasion have been associated with skin and tissue necrosis.

DO NOT REMOVE PADDING. Cotton-type padding under the cast may be pulled out in bits and pieces if not covered by the turned-back stockinette. This is ill advised, for the padding aids immobilization and alleviates much of the uncomfortable sensation of the cast saw.

EXERCISE JOINT. The patient should be encouraged to move all the adjacent joints not immobilized by the cast. A patient in a long leg cast should exercise the hip joint and toes and one in a long arm cast his shoulder, thumb, and fingers.

Isometric exercises of the muscles immobilized by the cast may be important to maintain good muscular tone. These exercises, however, are not routine and must be advised only on the recommendation of the physician.

CAST REMOVAL
Reasons

The technical skill required to remove plaster casts is not difficult to acquire. The decision to take off a cast demands experienced judgment. Casts are removed and changed for a variety of reasons. The plaster may have become too loose; a surgical wound requires inspection and stitch removal; or the extent of fracture healing is to be determined by x-ray.

If a cast is to be bivalved or completely removed, specific instructions pertaining to the handling of the part must be obtained from the physician. Cast removal and consideration of limb protection after removal are inseparable. The instructions depend on the type of injury, time interval from injury, and the next step in treatment.

The machine

The cast cutter is an electric saw that oscillates a circular blade with fine teeth. The amplitude of motion is small and the teeth relatively dull. If the moving blade lightly touches the skin, the latter vibrates with the oscillation and no harm is done. If additional pressure is exerted, the skin

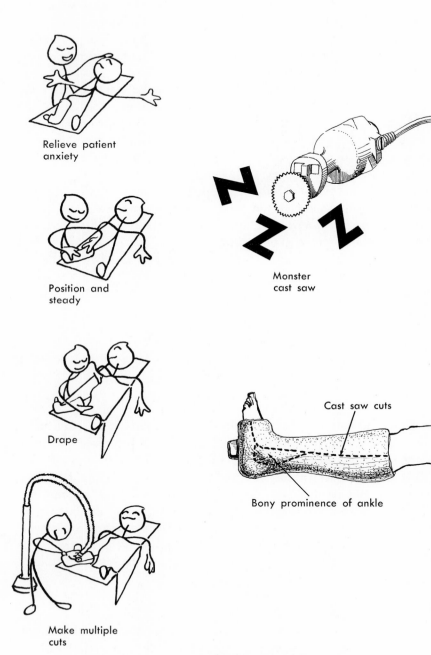

Relieve patient
anxiety

Position and
steady

Drape

Make multiple
cuts

Monster
cast saw

Cast saw cuts

Bony prominence of ankle

Fig. 9-6. Cast removal.

and subcutaneous tissues may be damaged. The saw readily cuts through the mature cast since it has no resiliency. The vibrations make the dust fly.

Relieve patient anxiety

The available cast cutter combines the harsh sounds of a dentist's drill and large vacuum cleaner. This ominous instrument transforms into an implement of destruction with a flip of the switch. Since a cast must be immobile for safe removal, the patient's confidence must be gained and his fears allayed so he will remain still. This is frequently no small task.

The patient should understand the saw's modus operandi and, if need be, have it demonstrated. Touching the moving blade lightly to the operator's hand is often helpful to indicate the harmlessness of the device. If the patient is a child, a similar demonstration on mother's palm will usually gain confidence. Mothers will usually submit to this ordeal despite their own anxiety to promote cooperation of the child (Fig. 9-6).

Technique of cast removal

The cast is steadied in an easily accessible position for the operator. The cast cutter is held in the major hand with the four fingers about the handle. The thumb touches the plaster before the blade and acts as a guard. The saw is gently but firmly pushed against and through the plaster in one place until there is a slight give. Too deep a penetration is prevented by the thumb. The tactile sensation of "being through" must become second nature (Fig. 9-7). When the blade is through, it is retracted and the cast divided immediately adjacent. The long cuts on a cast are made by repetitive penetration through the plaster in sequence. The cast cutter should not be run

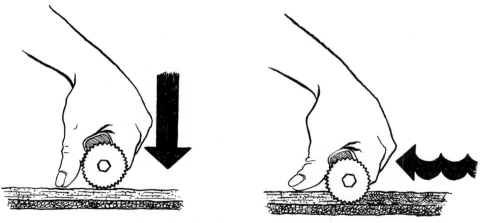

Fig. 9-7. Cast removal technique.

up and down a long area without being completely through in any one area. This uncontrolled handling will occasionally allow the saw to penetrate plaster in a reckless fashion, injuring the skin.

The method of cast saw use is the same for bivalving, windowing, or wedging. If a plaster surrounds a bony prominence and is difficult to remove or if the cast must be removed without disturbing the part, multiple cuts at various angles will be of benefit.

A "green" plaster is more difficult to cut with the saw, for the material is less rigid and the sensation of being through less secure. The blood-soaked bandage under a cast may pose similar problems.

The removal of "somebody else's" cast has a particular hazard. Some operators apply skintight plaster of Paris with minimal or no padding. Great caution must be exercised in the removal of such a plaster to prevent damage to the underlying tissues.

Cast removal requires caution and patience. Don't cause a cast saw burn!

CHAPTER 10

UPPER EXTREMITY CASTS

SHORT ARM CAST (SAC)

DESCRIPTION. The short arm cast extends distally from the proximal fore-arm to include the palm and the dorsum of the hand. The plaster completely covers the forearm but does not restrict elbow joint motion. The metacar-pophalangeal joints have complete motion, for the cast ends proximal to the distal palmar crease and the knuckles (Fig. 10-1).

This cast only partially immobilizes the wrist joint because the joints above and below are free. Pronation and supination of the forearm are not controlled.

APPLICATION. The patient is supine and the affected arm rests on the cast table with the elbow flexed to 90 degrees. The thumb and fingers are steadied by an assistant, with the wrist placed in the desired amount of dorsiflexion, palmar flexion, and ulnar or radial deviation. Pronation and supination are also controlled from the hand. Extreme positions of the joints should be avoided.

Additional padding is applied to the ulnar styloid. This is required partic-ularly with rotational motion in the cast.

The plaster is molded snugly to the palm and dorsum of the hand. A gentle anteroposterior mold is placed on the forearm.

The cast is trimmed proximally to permit complete elbow joint motion. The plaster is removed distally to allow 90 degrees of flexion at the distal palmar crease and to prevent irritation or rubbing on the knuckles. The plaster frequently is heaped up and becomes too thick in the thumb web and must be trimmed to allow pinch between the index finger and thumb.

INDICATIONS. Indications for a short arm cast include stable sprains of the wrist joint and stable fractures of the finger metacarpals, carpal bones, and distal radius (torus fractures in children, undisplaced styloid in adults).

SHORT ARM CAST WITH FINGER SPLINT

DESCRIPTION. A short arm cast has either an aluminum or Böhler finger splint incorporated into the plaster in the palm. The splint is fashioned to accept the finger "in the position of function." The finger is firmly held to the splint with adhesive tape. The tape is not sufficiently tight to cause constriction of the circulation or excessive pressure of the finger against the splint.

This device immobilizes the fingers and respective metacarpals.

INDICATIONS. Indications for this cast include phalangeal fractures, un-

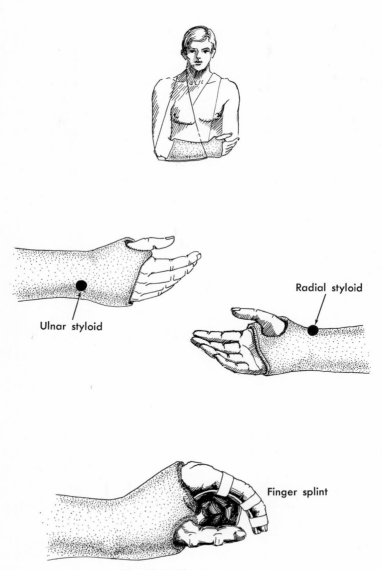

Fig. 10-1. Short arm cast.

stable finger metacarpal fractures, and ligamentous injuries to phalangeal and metacarpal phalangeal joints.

THUMB SPICA

DESCRIPTION. The thumb spica is a short arm cast including the thumb. "Spica" refers to the figure-eight or spiral of the bandages at the junction of distal and proximal portions of a cast. This type of bandaging occurs between the thumb and the hand. The cast extends distally on the thumb beyond the distal joint, exposing just the tip.

The thumb spica immobilizes the thumb metacarpal and phalanges. This cast decreases mobility of the wrist joint, primarily of the radial carpal bones, that is, the navicular and the greater and lesser multangular.

APPLICATION. The patient assumes the same position as for the application of a short arm cast. The thumb is placed in line with the long axis of the forearm (neutral) or the desired degrees of abduction and extension. The injury will determine the preferred position. If the position permits apposition of the index finger and thumb, the immobilized extremity will be more useful.

The molding of the cast is similar to a short arm cast with additional modeling of the thumb web and thumb.

Two-inch splints are useful in reinforcing the "spica" junction primarily on the radial side of the plaster.

INDICATIONS. Thumb spica casts may be used in fractures of the thumb metacarpal and phalanges, ligamentous injuries to the thumb joints, and fractures of the carpal navicular.

SUGAR TONG CAST

DESCRIPTION. A sugar tong cast is a single set of plaster splints extending from just proximal to the knuckles up the dorsal forearm, snugly wrapping about the distal humerus and coursing distally down the volar forearm to the distal palmar crease. The grip of the sugar tong is maintained by a circumferential wrap of bias stockinette or Ace bandages. If applied following an acute injury, the constriction from a circular plaster is avoided. After the postinjury swelling has subsided, the grip of the sugar tong may be tightened by snugly rewrapping the outer layer, providing better immobilization (Fig. 10-2).

This device partially immobilizes the wrist joint and restricts pronation and supination more effectively than the short arm cast.

APPLICATION. The splint is most easily applied with the patient supine, the arm resting on the cast table, and the hand controlled by an assistant with the elbow at 90 degrees of flexion.

Additional padding is placed over the bony prominences of the medial and lateral epicondyles of the distal humerus.

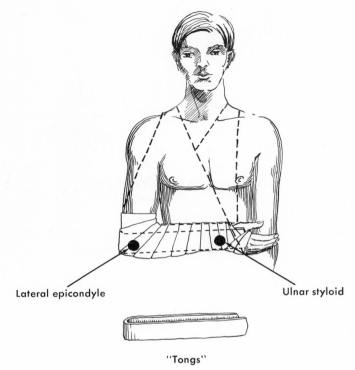

Lateral epicondyle   Ulnar styloid

"Tongs"

Fig. 10-2. Sugar tong cast.

The splints are molded to the palm and dorsum of the hand, to the forearm, and around the elbow. Excessive pressure is avoided at the area of the medial epicondyle to protect the ulnar nerve.

INDICATIONS. Sugar tong casts are used to immobilize fractures of the distal radius (Colles' fracture).

LONG ARM CAST (LAC)

DESCRIPTION. A long arm cast extends distally from the uppermost portion of the arm to include the palm and dorsum of the hand. The elbow joint is thus incorporated into the cast. The plaster comes to within 1 or 2 inches of the axilla medially but may extend farther proximally, anteriorly, posteriorly, and laterally. Finger, thumb, and shoulder joint motion are free (Fig. 10-3).

This cast provides excellent immobilization of the forearm and is superior to a short arm cast in restricting wrist joint motion, for pronation and supination are prevented. Partial immobilization is afforded the elbow joint and distal humerus.

APPLICATION. The cast is applied with the patient lying supine on the

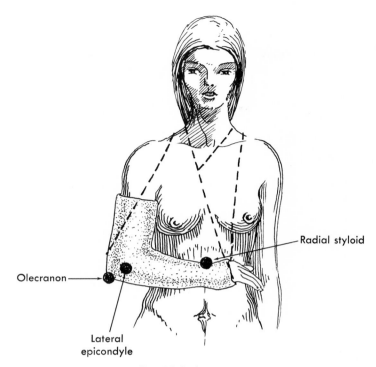

Olecranon

Lateral
epicondyle

Radial styloid

Fig. 10-3. Long arm cast.

cast table and the entire upper extremity suspended by an assistant. The patient's trunk should be flush with the side of the table so that the entire upper extremity is free. The elbow is usually positioned at 90 degrees of flexion with the desired amount of pronation or supination of the forearm. The patient's arm should be relaxed during application.

The ulnar styloid, olecranon, and medial and lateral epicondyles of the humerus require additional padding.

The cast may be applied as one unit, or the short arm portion may be wrapped first and, after "setting," extended up the arm. Application and molding of the plaster in the antecubital fossa must not constrict the neurovascular structures in this area. Binding will occur if elbow flexion increases with the preset plaster in place, and therefore motion must be prevented during application. The cast should fit the arm snugly with gentle molding in the anteroposterior plane to alleviate any pressure on the neurovascular structures as they leave the axilla through the proximal medial arm.

Plaster splints are optional to reinforce the posterior cast and to increase strength at the elbow joint while decreasing the amount of circular plaster in the antecubital fossa.

The fingers and thumb are trimmed free, like a short arm cast. The proximal portion of the cast must be trimmed medially 1 to 2 inches from the axilla to prevent neurovascular compression.

INDICATIONS. Indications for a long arm cast include unstable ligamentous injuries of the wrist joint, unstable fractures of the carpal bones, fractures of one or both bones of the forearm, stable injuries of the elbow joint, and stable fractures of the distal humerus.

HANGING ARM CAST

DESCRIPTION. A hanging arm cast is a long arm circular plaster suspended by a bandage extending around the patient's neck and attached to the superior aspect of the cast at the wrist joint. The weight of the cast applies continuous gentle traction to the humerus with the patient standing or sitting. The neck strap supports some of the cast's weight and stabilizes the traction forces. The arm portion of the plaster does not extend as far proximally as a usual long arm cast (Fig. 10-4).

The hanging cast does not immobilize the joint above or the joint below a fractured humerus. The effectiveness of this apparatus is dependent on the traction forces. The patient treated with a hanging arm cast is advised to remain erect or semierect at all times to provide the necessary traction. At night the patient must sleep in the sitting position.

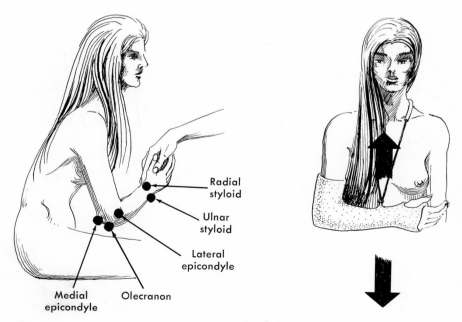

Radial
styloid

Ulnar
styloid

Lateral
epicondyle

Medial
epicondyle

Olecranon

Fig. 10-4. Hanging arm cast.

APPLICATION. The hanging arm cast is applied with the patient sitting and flexed forward at the waist, permitting the arm to hang freely in front of the trunk. The forearm is suspended by an assistant holding the fingers and thumb with the elbow flexed to 90 degrees and the forearm in the desired rotation. In this position all sides of the extremity may be reached and gentle traction is applied by the distal humerus and forearm.

The needs for padding and cautions in plaster application are the same as a long arm cast. The hanging arm cast is purposely made lighter to prevent excessive traction at the fracture site and possible distraction. The cast does not extend as far proximally on the arm as the long arm cast. The exact distance varies with personal preference but in general is to approximately the midportion.

The positioning of the attachment of the neck sling to the set cast partially controls fracture angulation of the humerus. Dorsal placement of this force at the wrist tends to align the distal fragment in valgus. A volar attachment places a varus stress on the distal fragment. The neck sling is attached to the superior surface of the cast by plaster or metallic loops incorporated into the cast.

INDICATIONS. Hanging arm casts are used for spiral or comminuted fracture of humeral shaft and displaced fractures of the surgical neck of the humerus.

VELPEAU DRESSING OR SLING AND SWATHE

DESCRIPTION. The Velpeau dressing or sling and swathe is a cloth or plaster bandage that splints the arm to the chest with the elbow in flexion and the forearm against the abdomen. The types of dressings vary, but all include a circumferential wrap of arm to the chest and sling-type support to the forearm.

This bandage immobilizes the shoulder girdle to include the scapula, clavicle, and humerus as well as their mutual joints. Fixation of the humerus is not rigid if elbow joint motion is permitted. The humerus is immobilized in internal rotation when the forearm is splinted anteriorly to the trunk.

APPLICATION. The bandage is applied with the patient sitting and the unaffected arm placed on the top of his head.

The following Velpeau type dressing is satisfactory; however, other varieties are equally effective. The upper extremity is placed in a triangular cloth sling affixed around the neck. This supports the forearm with the elbow flexed. The forearm may be raised or lowered, increasing or decreasing elbow flexion by tightening or loosening the sling at the neck. The proper level is usually the position of comfort for the arm. The sling behind the neck is more comfortable if pinned rather than knotted, which leaves a wad to irritate the skin. The free lateral corner of the sling is folded and pinned anteriorly to itself, providing additional support to the elbow. The sling is adjusted to avoid skin-to-skin contact of the arm or forearm to the trunk.

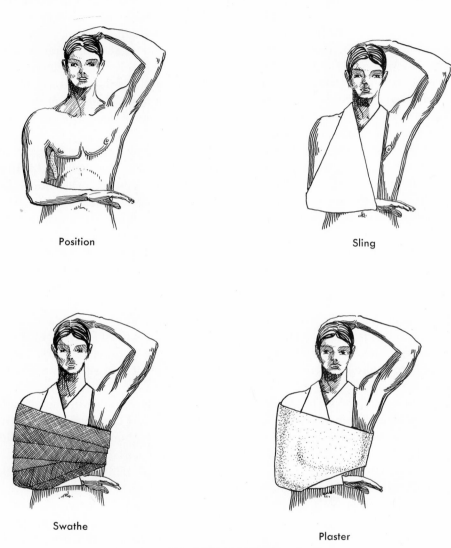

Position

Sling

Swathe

Plaster

Fig. 10-5. Velpeau bandage.

Prolonged contact of these surfaces leads to skin irritation and maceration. Cotton type padding is placed high in the axilla to absorb perspiration. Dusting powders are not recommended for this purpose. Bias-cut stockinette is then wrapped circumferentially around the trunk and arm, coursing above and below the wrist and leaving the hand free. Additional support for the elbow may be obtained by carrying the stockinette under the elbow and over the shoulder. Care should be exercised during application to prevent pressure on the ulnar nerve at the medial epicondyle. The bias-cut stockinette must be safety-pinned in many places to the underlying sling to prevent sliding of stockinette and ultimate dishevelment. Plaster of Paris rolls and splints applied and molded over the Velpeau will reinforce and make the dressing more secure (Fig. 10-5).

This type of dressing places skin surfaces in immediate contact and encloses them. Skin care is impossible and superficial irritation is common. The dressing should be changed frequently and rarely left on continuously for more than 3 or 4 weeks.

The Velpeau bandage may not be satisfactory in a female with large breasts. The large skin surfaces and the configuration of the lateral chest are best sidestepped and another form of immobilization used.

INDICATIONS. Velpeau dressings are used to treat fractures of the scapula, clavicle, and humerus; acromioclavicular joint injuries; and ligamentous injuries to the shoulder joint.

CHAPTER 11

LOWER EXTREMITY CASTS

SHORT LEG NON—WEIGHT-BEARING CAST (SLNWBC)

DESCRIPTION. The short leg cast extends from just below the knee joint distally to the base of the toes. The plantar surface of the plaster is often carried beyond the toes, providing support and protection in the form of a toe plate. Knee joint motion is full; however, flexion of the toes may be restricted by the volar plate.

The ankle joint and metatarsal shafts are only partially immobilized by this cast, for the joints above or below these structures are free. The bones and intervening joints of the hind and midfoot are more rigidly immobilized.

APPLICATION. This cast may be applied with the patient in a number of positions, depending on personal preference. The patient may be sitting on the edge of the cast table with the leg dependent and the toes steadied by an assistant. If the patient is prone, the knee is flexed to 90 degrees and the leg controlled by the toes. In the supine position, the leg is supported and held still proximally under the partially flexed knee and distally by the toes. The last position is most convenient to the operator. However, it requires the assistant to hold the weight of the leg during the complete application. In each instance, the placement of the toes determines the degree of equinus or plantar flexion of the ankle and the degree of eversion or inversion of the foot. Once the leg is placed in the desired position and stabilized, continuous vigilance must prevent any change in position. Most short leg casts are applied with the ankle joint at 90 degrees and without eversion or inversion of the heel. Additional padding is advised over the neck of the fibula to prevent compression of the peroneal nerve. The bony prominences of the medial and lateral malleoli should receive increased protection against pressure. The "setting" plaster is molded around both malleoli and on either side of the Achilles tendon. The cast should conform to the non—weight-bearing longitudinal arch of the foot. Special molding on the leg is not necessary. The cast is often reinforced at the posterior ankle by a set of splints from the posterior leg extending to the plantar surface of the foot. The cast is trimmed proximally sufficiently to permit complete knee joint motion. Distally, the plaster should allow complete extension of the toes. The cast must support at least the metatarsal heads. Plantar support at the toes is indicated with certain injuries and is routine for certain operators.

INDICATIONS. This short leg cast is used to treat stable ankle fractures; stable ligamentous ankle joint injuries; fractures of the calcaneus, talus, navicular, cuboid, and cuneiforms; subluxations and dislocations of the tarsal bones; and stable fractures of the metacarpals.

SHORT LEG WEIGHT-BEARING CAST (SLWBC)

DESCRIPTION. The short leg weight-bearing cast is a short leg cast with a walking heel or iron on the plantar surface (Fig. 11-1).

APPLICATION. The special techniques and precautions for a short leg cast are applied. The walking heel is applied after the cast has completely

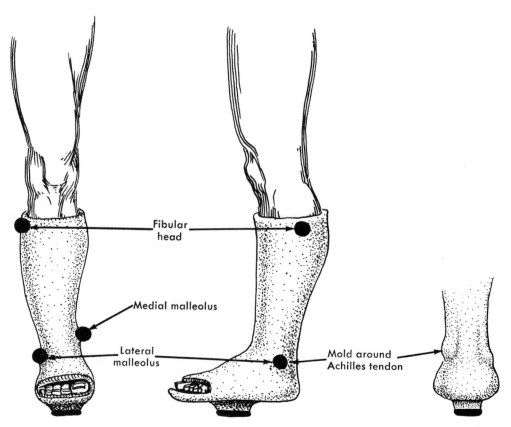

Fig. 11-1. Short leg weight-bearing cast.

reached the "green stage." This delay prevents indentation of the sole of the cast by this device. The molded plantar arch surface is converted to a flat platform by additional plaster splints. The heel is placed in the midline in the sagittal plane, and the center of its weight-bearing surface is in line with the anterior border of the cast. If the heel is placed more posteriorly, the toes hit the ground during ambulation and the patient automatically externally rotates the cast during weight bearing to prevent this impingement. This maneuver places unnecessary rotary stress on the immobilized structures. The heel is held to the cast by additional plaster rolls around the ankle and foot, and gaps between the former and the sole are filled by pushing in tucks and folds of splints and the securing wrap.

INDICATIONS. Indications are the same as for a short leg non–weight-bearing cast.

PATELLAR TENDON WEIGHT-BEARING CAST (PTWBC)

DESCRIPTION. The "patty-bear" cast is a short leg walking cast with additional proximal support provided by molding over the tibial condylar flare, femoral condyles, patellar tendon, and popliteal space. The top of the cast extends from the middle of the patella in front posteriorly above the femoral condyles and then distally to approximately 1 inch below the popliteal crease. The lower dimensions of the plaster are identical with a short leg cast (Fig. 11-2).

This plaster does not immobilize the joint above and the joint below the leg. However, it effectively transmits applied weight above a fracture and controls proximal and distal rotation by snug molding. This method of immobilization has proved its value.

APPLICATION. The patient sits on the edge of the cast table with the leg dependent and the ankle held in neutral position by an assistant. A minimum of padding—only one layer of stockinette increased at the malleoli and neck of the fibula by Webril—is advised. The cast is applied in three sections to allow sufficient time for precise molding of each part. Plaster is first applied to the foot and ankle and worked until the "green stage" has been reached. The cast is then extended proximally to below the level of the tibial tubercle and molded snugly to the anterior tibial surface, the anterior muscular compartment, and the calf. The triangular configuration of the plaster controls rotation. The third section of the cast is applied just prior to the second reaching the "green stage" and with the knee held in 45 degrees instead of 90 degrees of flexion. The plaster is molded to the medial and lateral flares of the tibial condyles, transversely across the patellar tendon, and around the femoral condyles. After setting, the front of the cast is cut down to the inferior pole of the patella; however, the extensions around the femoral condyles are preserved to prevent rotation. The back of

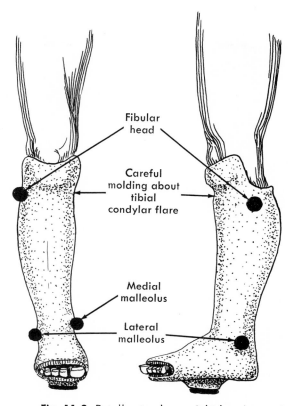

Fibular
head

Careful
molding about
tibial
condylar flare

Medial
malleolus

Lateral
malleolus

Fig. 11-2. Patellar tendon weight-bearing cast.

the cast is trimmed to ensure complete knee flexion. A walking heel is positioned and applied in the usual manner.

INDICATIONS. The patellar tendon cast is used for unstable fractures of the tibia and fibula.

LONG LEG CAST (LLC)

DESCRIPTION. The long leg cast extends the short leg cast proximally to include the knee joint and thigh. The top of the plaster should reach the groin and the bottom the base of the toes.

The cast adequately immobilizes the leg, ankle joint, and hindfoot but is not sufficient for protection of unstable injuries of the distal femur or knee joint.

APPLICATION. This plaster requires two stages. A short leg cast is applied with the patient supine as previously described and allowed to "set." The assistant then holds the hardened short leg cast with the knee joint in the desired position, and the plaster is extended to the upper thigh.

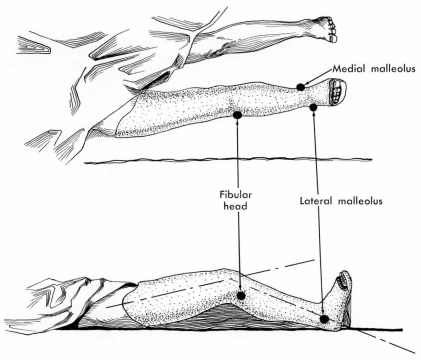

Fig. 11-3. Long leg cast.

The knee is usually placed in 15 to 20 degrees of flexion to relax the ligaments joining the femur to the tibia. If the knee joint is in complete extension, these ligaments are taut and motion of the femur is transmitted to the proximal tibia. Additional padding is occasionally recommended over the front of the patella. The plaster on the thigh is firmly molded in the shape of a quadrilateral socket to prevent rotation. The cast is also shaped just above the superior border of the patella in the form of a horseshoe with the convexity proximal. The medial and lateral aspects of the knee joint are reinforced with sets of splints for increased strength. Trimming of the bottom of the cast is identical with the short leg cast. Proximally, the plaster should be left as high as possible to ensure the maximum grip on the thigh (Fig. 11-3).

INDICATIONS. Long leg casts are used for unstable fractures of the tibia and fibula, unstable fractures and fracture-dislocations of the ankle joint, and stable injuries to the knee joint and distal femur.

LONG LEG WEIGHT-BEARING CAST (LLWBC)

The long leg weight-bearing cast is a long leg cast with a walking heel. The application and indications are similar to the long leg cast.

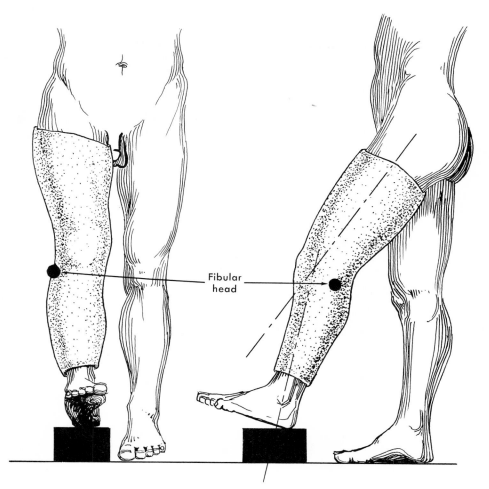

Fig. 11-4. Long leg cylinder cast.

LONG LEG CYLINDER CAST (LLCC)

DESCRIPTION. The long leg cylinder cast extends from the upper thigh to just above the flare of the medial and lateral malleoli.

The plaster partially immobilizes the distal femur, knee joint, and proximal tibia.

APPLICATION. The cast is applied either with the patient supine and the lower extremity supported by the heel or with the patient standing on the uninjured leg and the other supported by the foot on a low footstool or rest. The former method may utilize one or two stages, depending on the desired position of the knee joint. If flexion is indicated, this attitude is more satisfactorily obtained by applying the lower portion of the cast first with support under the heel. The plaster is completed after this section has set. The knee is controlled by holding the hardened cast. The second method allows the application of the entire cast simultaneously with control of the knee joint position. The areas of the malleoli, proximal fibula, and kneecap may require increased protective padding (Fig. 11-4). The general conical shape of the thigh and calf with the apex located distally permits the cylinder cast to slide down the leg. This slippage may be prevented in part by skin adhesives and tapes. However, it is best controlled by snug molding and, if indicated, a partially flexed knee. Quadrilaterally molding the thigh and a "horseshoe" over the patella is indicated. The cast is strengthened at the knee joint by lateral sets of splints. The cast is trimmed distally to prevent any irritation at the malleoli.

INDICATIONS. The long leg cylinder cast is applied to stable injuries to the distal femur, knee joint, or proximal tibia.

CHAPTER 12

BODY CASTS

GENERAL CONSIDERATIONS

The cervical, thoracic, and lumbar spines are immobilized to permit repair of unstable injuries, healing of surgical spinal fusions, and symptomatic relief from degenerative conditions. Absolutely rigid fixation of either the cervical, thoracic, or lumbar spines cannot be achieved by plaster because the chest must move with respiration and the abdomen must vary in size with eating. Adequate immobilization is possible by certain anatomic areas utilizing points of fixation controlling motion of the whole. These points of fixation are created by careful molding to and around specific bony surfaces.

MINERVA JACKET

DESCRIPTION. The Minerva jacket is an ambulatory plaster cast immobilizing the cervical spine. The plaster extends from the frontal and occipital scalp areas caudally to cover the neck, chest, and iliac crests. The ears and face are exposed, and the upper extremities have full motion through windows at the shoulder (Fig. 12-1).

APPLICATION

Positioning. This cast is applied with the patient standing or sitting. The recumbent position, even with the use of a fracture table, is not satisfactory.

If the patient has been in bed for a prolonged period just prior to cast application, the erect position may cause dizziness and fainting. The patient must be observed for symptoms and signs to anticipate and avoid a collapse.

When changing from the supine to the erect position, the patient is moved as a unit with the head, neck, and trunk rigid. This move requires sufficient help.

The head and neck must be stabilized in both the standing and sitting positions. This is accomplished primarily by the patient's muscles but is

119

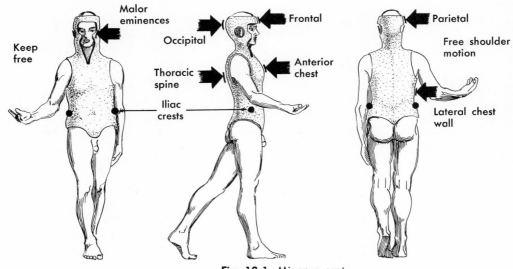

Fig. 12-1. Minerva cast.

often assisted by previously placed skeletal skull tongs through which gentle vertical traction is applied. The cloth head halter is not advised, for it prevents precise molding. The patient steadies himself by holding fixed objects (such as intravenous poles) with each hand. Before starting the cast, the patient must be comfortable and stable.

Padding. An 8- to 10-inch stockinette is placed over the head, neck, and trunk, with holes cut laterally for the arms and a small opening over the nose for ventilation. The stockinette is pinned on the top of the head to prevent sliding and cut about the neck to correct the wrinkling and bunching. This initial underpadding protects the eyes during plaster application and is convenient to turn over and smooth the edges on completion.

The tubular stockinette is then covered with two layers of cotton padding. The ears may be covered with small cups to identify their exact location for subsequent trimming. Felt pads are often placed over the iliac crests superficial to the cotton to additionally protect these areas. The felt pads will not slide if the plaster is applied directly over them.

Points of fixation and molding. Immobilization in the sagittal plane is by fixation to the forehead, malar eminences, sternum, and pubic symphysis anteriorly and the occiput, thoracic, and lumbar spines in back. Lateral motion is prevented by controlling the head above the ears, the lateral chest walls, and the pelvis just below the iliac crests. Rotation of the head is limited by molding over the malar eminences. The weight of the cast is supported on the iliac crests. The finished cast should have gentle indentation superior to and gripping the crests.

Plaster of Paris rolls are applied initially to define the limits of the cast. Multiple splints of varying sizes are then used to reinforce the forehead and occiput, malar eminences, posterior neck, shoulders, and trunk. Plaster rolls hold the splints in place and smooth the surface. Sufficiently rapid plaster application requires two operators working with dexterity. As the plaster sets, the points of fixation are continuously molded to ensure a snug fit. The molding must continue until the "green stage" has been reached, which requires the operator's perseverance.

Trimming. The excess plaster is removed with either a cast saw or a knife. The former is recommended for areas close to the ears, eyes, and throat.

The cast above the level of the forehead and occiput contributes no fixation and is removed for ventilation. The ears are completely exposed to prevent any impingement with resultant discomfort. The face is trimmed from the eyebrows distally around the eyes, maintaining the malar eminences as points of fixation. Below this level the cast swings laterally around the jaw and forms a V-neck over the anterior chest. The configuration of plaster holds the skull rigid but permits the jaw to move freely in eating. The latter cannot be used as a point of fixation. The plaster is trimmed at the shoulders to allow complete shoulder joint motion. The bottom of the cast is removed proximally from each groin to permit comfortable sitting with the thighs flexed, but it is left over the pubic area for fixation. Laterally, the plaster is trimmed above the greater trochanters to allow for their motion but remains snugly around the iliac crests. The back of the cast is brought to the upper end of the anal crease. After trimming, the stockinette is turned over the rough cast edges and attached to the outer surface of the plaster.

If skeletal tongs have been used, these are removed and the wounds dressed.

BODY JACKET

DESCRIPTION. The body jacket extends from the upper chest down over the trunk to the pubis and covers the iliac crests. Shoulder and hip joint motion are complete.

The body jacket does not provide rigid immobilization but rather supports and partially controls motion in the thoracic and lumbar spines. To more adequately immobilize the thoracic spine with plaster, the cervical spine must be included. Similarly, the thighs and pelvis should be included if motion in the lumbar spine is to be substantially diminished. The partial immobilization provided by the cast is, however, often sufficient (Fig. 12-2).

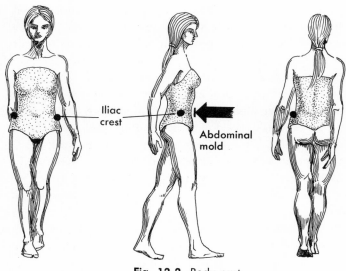

Fig. 12-2. Body cast.

APPLICATION

Positioning. Body jackets are applied with the patient standing, sitting, supine, or prone. The erect positions promote a better fitting cast, particularly if the patient is to be ambulatory. Casts fitted in the recumbent positions tend to shift when the patient becomes upright.

If the plaster is applied with the patient standing or sitting, he stabilizes his trunk by holding to fixed objects. The lumbar spine may be in flexion, neutral, or in extension.

The prone position with the spine in extension is used most frequently to apply the cast. The patient is suspended between two tables with the head, shoulders, and upper extremities on one and the thighs and lower extremities on the other. The desired degree of extension is obtained by choosing the appropriate table heights and altering the distances between the tables. This position leaves the trunk completely exposed for wrapping and molding. The patient must necessarily be comfortable and completely secured prior to plaster application.

If the supine position is indicated, the patient lies on a taut canvas strap measuring 6 inches in width. The latter is attached to two ends of a fracture table and is under sufficient tension so that it does not give under the patient's body weight. The strap runs longitudinally and supports the back of the head, thoracic and lumbar spines, and buttocks. The lower extremities require additional support. A portion of strap is covered during cast application. This is removed from either end when the cast is "set," the strap detached from the fracture table, and the patient supported on another surface. The patient must be securely stabilized prior to applying the cast.

Padding. Tubular stockinette, cotton padding, and felt pads are placed in a routine manner.

Points of fixation and molding. Flexion and extension are restricted by cast fixation over the sternum, symphysis pubis, and thoracolumbar spine. Immobilization in the frontal plane is the result of a snug plaster mold over the lateral chest walls and the iliac crests. Rotation is controlled by the combination of all of these. The cast weight rests on the iliac crests.

The cast is applied using a combination of rolls and splints. In addition to continuously molding over the points of fixation, the abdomen should be moderately compressed if the cast is applied in the erect position. This molding increases support to the lumbar spine.

Trimming. The cast should be trimmed down to permit free shoulder motion but still maintain fixation to the upper sternum and thoracic spine. The bottom of the cast has the same configuration as a Minerva jacket.

CHAPTER 13

SPICA CASTS

GENERAL CONSIDERATIONS

A spica cast immobilizes an appendage to the main part. The shoulder and hip spica casts immobilize the upper and lower extremities, respectively, to the trunk.

SHOULDER SPICA CAST

DESCRIPTION. The shoulder spica combines a long arm cast and a body jacket. The entire upper extremity is immobilized with the exception of thumb and fingers and joined to a body cast at the shoulder (Fig. 13-1).

This plaster effectively immobilizes the shoulder girdle, arm, and elbow joint.

APPLICATION. The patient may be erect or supine.

In the upright position the long arm and body cast are usually applied separately and then joined at the shoulder. This two-stage approach permits better control of the upper extremity during long arm cast application and ease in positioning the arm to the "set" body cast. If the cast is applied supine, the patient's head and thoracolumbar spine are supported by a taut canvas strap or "slippery stick," with the affected upper extremity suspended by the thumb and fingers. The trunk and legs assume the same stance as for the application of a supine body jacket. The position of the arm and the relationship of upper extremity to trunk can be maintained, and thus the entire cast is applied as one unit. The strap or stick is removed after the cast has "set." The patient's position on the apparatus must be secure and comfortable.

The requirements for padding are those of the long arm cast and body cast.

Plaster application is routine, with the exception that the shoulder joint must be reinforced to support the long lever arm of the upper extremity. Additional plaster of Paris splints may not be sufficient to prevent breakage. The "plastered" arm and trunk form two sides of a triangle that may be completed by a stick extending from the elbow or forearm

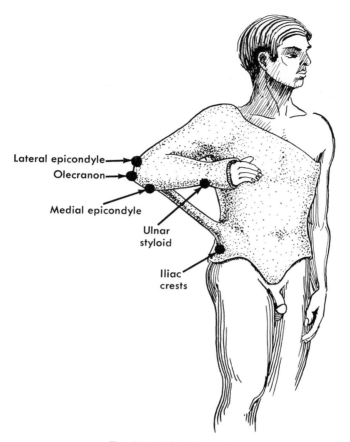

Lateral epicondyle

Olecranon

Medial epicondyle

Ulnar
styloid

Iliac
crests

Fig. 13-1. Shoulder spica cast.

to the region of the iliac crest and incorporated into the cast. The completion of the triangle markedly enhances the cast strength at the shoulder joint. The wooden strut is positioned and incorporated after the cast has set to prevent indentations of the plaster.

INDICATIONS. The shoulder spica cast is used for unstable fractures of the shoulder girdle and humerus, dislocations of the shoulder girdle, and unstable elbow joint injuries.

HIP SPICA CASTS

DESCRIPTION. Hip spica casts immobilize one or both lower extremities to the trunk. The single hip spica includes the trunk and one lower extremity; the one and one-half hip spica in addition immobilizes the other lower extremity to the knee; and the double hip spica joins two long leg casts to a body jacket. The upper part of the casts extends to just below the nipple line. The degree of immobilization indicated dictates whether one or both legs are included.

Hip joint motion is not completely restricted by a single hip spica cast. Movement of the pelvis in this plaster is possible and is transferred to the enclosed hip joint. If the opposite thigh is included (one and one-half hip spica), rotation of the pelvis is limited and the restriction of hip joint motion is more adequate. To immobilize "the joint above and joint below," a femoral shaft fracture necessarily requires a one and one-half hip spica cast. The double hip spica cast immobilizes both hip joints and femoral shafts by controlling the pelvis proximally and the knees distally.

Double hip spica for congenital dislocation of the hip

Unilateral and bilateral congenital dislocations of the hip are immobilized in double hip spica casts. This cast is applied following closed or open reduction of the dislocation and after reconstructive surgery to improve the anatomic relation of the hip joint.

APPARATUS AND POSITIONING. The cast is applied supine on a special apparatus consisting of a seat plate to support the buttocks, a perineal post against which the pelvis is stabilized, and a movable platform upon which the upper trunk and head are rested. The distance between the saddle and the platform is varied depending on the size of the child.

The patient's buttocks are placed on the seat plate with the lower extremities controlled just below the knees by an assistant and the perineum positioned against the post. The upper trunk rests on the platform, leaving the abdomen, lumbar spine, lower thoracic spine, and chest exposed. The upper body and extremities are controlled by an additional assistant. The lower extremities are usually immobilized in one of two positions. The first is the frog leg or 90-90-90, in which the hips are abducted to 90 degrees and completely externally rotated, with knees flexed to 90 degrees and the ankles in neutral (Fig. 13-2). The second position places the hips in 40 to 60 degrees of abduction and moderate internal rotation, with the knees straight and the ankles in neutral.

PADDING. Tubular stockinette is recommended next to the skin to cover the trunk and lower extremities. This material is turned over the completed cast to smooth the edges and prevent crumbling. A removable pad (small towel or folded stockinette) is placed under the tubular stockinette over the abdomen. This "belly pad" increases the size of the cast in this area and anticipates the marked increase in stomach size that occurs in babies after feeding. The remainder of the padding is routine, with attention to the bony prominences of the trunk and lower extremities.

APPLICATION. The plaster and also final underpadding are applied first

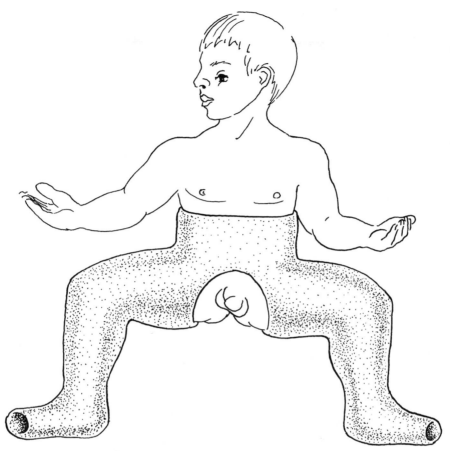

Fig. 13-2. Frog-legged spica for hip dislocation.

to the trunk and lower extremities to just below the knees. The desired position of the hips and knees is maintained by holding the proximal legs. The additional plaster splints required to reinforce the front and back of the hip joints are incorporated with circular rolls. The plaster should be carefully molded to prevent any pressure over the abdomen. When the first portion of the cast has set, the remainder of padding and plaster is applied with the legs and ankles controlled in the desired positions by the toes. If the amount of knee flexion changes, the leg may impinge on the set cast; this must be watched for and avoided. The cast should be carried beyond the tips of the toes to subsequently protect these digits. After the entire cast has set, the patient is taken off the table by removing the perineal post and slipping out the saddle. If the cast is placed on a good-sized child, a wooden crossbar between the legs will increase strength and prevent cracking at the hip joints.

TRIMMING. The top of the cast is trimmed down to just below the nipple line and around the chest. The width of the exposed perineal area between the thighs is approximately four fingers wide and extends from the symphysis pubis in front to the proximal anal crease in back. The size of this area must be adequate for diapering, yet not weaken the cast or permit the buttock and thighs to protrude excessively.

Adult hip spica cast

The single, one and one-half, and double hip spica casts immobilize injuries and reconstructive surgeries of the pelvis, hip joint, femur, and

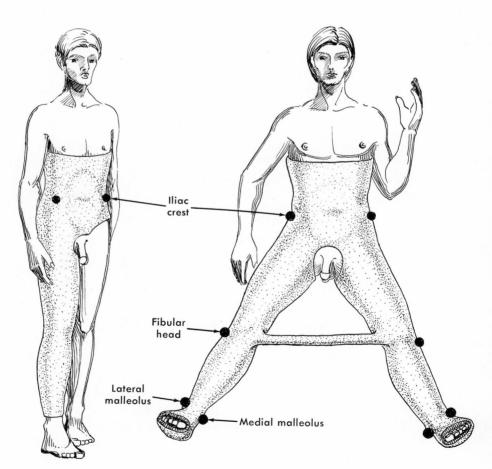

Iliac crest

Fibular head

Lateral malleolus

Medial malleolus

Fig. 13-3. Single and double adult hip spica.

occasionally the knee. The selection of the specific cast is determined by the amount of the immobilization required (Fig. 13-3).

APPARATUS AND POSITIONING. Hip spica casts are usually applied with the patient supine on a fracture table. The fracture tables vary depending on the commercial manufacturer; however, they all have certain features in common. There is a saddle and perineal post to support the buttocks and steady the pelvis, stirrups to hold the ankles and feet in the indicated position, and an adjustable platform upon which the upper trunk is rested. The seat plates come in different sizes, depending on the support required. The stirrups are designed to control the ankles and feet when the latter are secured. The foot pieces position the lower extremities in the indicated amount of abduction or adduction and may be adjusted to apply traction with the perineal post as countertraction. The legs and thighs may be supported by rests from the table below or suspended by slings from an overhead frame. The distance from the seat plate to the upper trunk rest is determined by the size of the patient. The fracture table should be set up and ready prior to accepting the patient.

The transfer of a patient from bed to fracture table requires adequate personnel. Concern for the patient's modesty must be shown by covering the sensitive areas. The injured part is controlled and guided by the physician to prevent possible damage. A trapeze on the bed or fracture table may permit the patient to assist in the move. The transfer is a combined effort of patient and personnel carried out in unison, with the patient's head, trunk, and upper and lower extremities controlled. The patient is positioned on the saddle and the perineal post inserted. The proximal platform is adjusted to support the upper trunk and head. The feet are firmly secured to the padded stirrups and the indicated support and traction applied to the lower extremities. With the patient in the desired position, the parts of the fracture table are tightened to prevent motion during plaster application.

PADDING. The use of tubular stockinette is recommended for patient comfort. Cotton padding is then applied, followed by additional protection to the iliac crest, sacrum (if the cast is non–weight bearing), and prominences of the lower extremities.

APPLICATION. Plaster rolls and splints are applied in the usual manner. The front, side, and back of the hip joint must be reinforced with sets of splints, for this area is under considerable stress. The cast is molded to the iliac crests, groin and buttocks, and lower extremities. The cast may be applied in sections for convenience, with additional reinforcements at the junctions. After the main portion of the cast has set, the feet are removed from the stirrups and included in the cast. A crossbar between the legs should be used with either the one and one-half or double spica cast to increase strength.

The patient's transfer back to bed also requires sufficient manpower. The move is carried out after removing the perineal post.

TRIMMING. The cast is removed to below the nipple level around the trunk. The perineal area is exposed to permit bowel and bladder function with proper personal hygiene. The thigh portion of the one and one-half hip spica should be trimmed enough to allow complete knee flexion.

Walking hip spica

The walking hip spica is a single hip spica either incorporating the foot or carried down to a level just above the malleoli. The immobilized thigh is usually in neutral position regarding abduction and adduction but may be in some flexion and external rotation.

The cast is applied with the patient standing on the elevated good leg or a fracture table. The former method obtains a better fit for ambulation.

Padding, plaster application, molding, and trimming follow the same rules for any hip spica. Reinforcement at the hip must be particularly strong, for a crossbar is not possible. If the foot is included, a walking heel is applied in the usual position.

CHAPTER 14

CIRCUMFERENTIAL TRACTION

GENERAL CONSIDERATIONS

Circumferential traction is useful in the management of a variety of orthopaedic diseases and injuries. The traction forces are not great but may be applied for a relatively long period of time. The forces act primarily to partially immobilize and only secondarily to distract.

The traction is applied by encircling devices that grip the skin of the head, trunk, or limb in regions having a larger circumference or bony prominences. The most commonly employed apparatus are the head halter for cervical spine traction and the pelvic belt for the lumbar spine (Fig. 14-1). Encircling devices employing traction are occasionally used to partially immobilize acute injuries to the extremities and to facilitate the patient's transfer. The latter application is not definitive treatment and should be used only temporarily.

The force applied through the apparatus is limited by the skin tolerance to pressure. This may not be exceeded or tissue necrosis will occur. Since the traction force is not usually large, countertraction is provided by the patient's body weight.

Circumferential traction apparatus requires a fixed or semifixed pulley system, usually with the patient sitting or recumbent in bed. The application of the encircling device and traction is swiftly and safely performed by the orthopaedic assistant. The latter should immediately remove the apparatus if any problems arise.

BED AND PULLEY SYSTEM

A standard hospital bed equipped with a frame to attach pulleys at specific fixed points is adequate. The bed should permit independent elevation of the head, knees, and feet. The pulley system consists of pulleys, rope, weight carriers, and weights. The type of pulley is less important than their proper placement to ensure the correct direction of the traction. The most satisfactory rope is $\frac{1}{8}$ inch in diameter, for it is easily tied and glides freely in the pulleys. The type of weight carrier

131

Pelvic belt

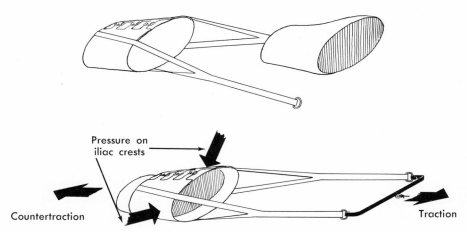

Fig. 14-1. Circumferential traction.

and weights are of no significance if they are securely attached to the rope and hang freely off the bed.

KNOTS *(Fig. 14-2)*

The ropes are secured to various parts of any traction by knots. Personal preference and need will dictate the types of knots used; they should be secure and not slip. The following three cover most contingencies.

BOWLINE. The bowline forms a fixed loop that will not slip. It is useful to hang some weight carriers.

TWO HALF-HITCHES. Two half-hitches firmly secure the rope to a ring or pole. The loop may be pulled tight but is easily loosened.

SQUARE KNOT. The square knot may be used to join two pieces of rope together and, if tied correctly, holds firmly.

Wrapping adhesive tape around the rope at the point to be cut will prevent unraveling. Taping the ends of the knots to make them more secure is optional.

HEAD HALTER TRACTION

INDICATIONS. Continuous gentle cervical spine traction applied by a head halter is useful in treating many cervical spine syndromes. Degenerative disk disease with or without nerve root impingement, cervical arthritis, and rarely cervical spine sprains are benefited by the partial immobilization and gentle distraction afforded.

Bowline

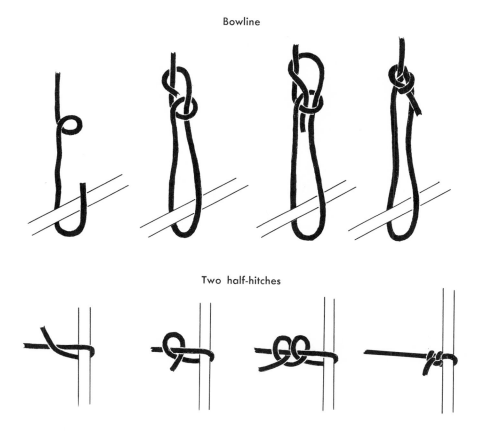

Two half-hitches

Square knot

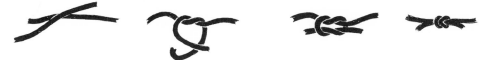

Fig. 14-2. Knots.

This traction has no place in the management of cervical spine fractures. Stable fractures should be more adequately immobilized with a collar or Minerva jacket. Unstable fractures should immediately be protected by the use of skeletal traction with skull tongs. The head halter does not provide sufficient protection to prevent displacement of the fracture with possible cord compression and paralysis.

APPARATUS AND APPLICATION. A head halter, spreader bar, and pulley system are required to place the patient in this traction. The head halter is usually made out of cloth or cloth-like material, with a broad flat surface posteriorly to fit the occiput and a lesser surface anteriorly to fit the chin. The occipital and chin pieces are slipped over the head and placed in their respective positions. The two surfaces are fitted to the head by joining and adjusting two lateral straps to the proper length. The occipital and chin pieces join on each side near the top of the head and end with a loop or ring to attach to the spreader bar. The spreader bar holds the sides of the head halter away from the face and is tied by rope to the pulley system.

Since head halter cervical spine traction is justified by the fact that it renders patient comfort, the operator should apply the apparatus without jerking or twisting the neck. This occurs if the head halter and spreader bar are applied initially and then the weights added. The appropriate directional pull should be determined and the pulley system set up accordingly and tied to the spreader bar. The weight of the pulley system is held while the spreader bar is attached to the head halter and then gradually released to the apparatus. This prevents jerking of the neck from rapid loading on the head halter. The traction force should also be removed in a considerate and deliberate fashion.

The maximum weight recommended for continuous traction is 5 pounds or less. A traction force greater than this creates more discomfort than it relieves.

POSITION. The traction force should place the cervical spine in a neutral or slightly flexed position. These two positions increase the size of the intervertebral foramina for the passage of the spinal nerves and relieve pressure on these structures. Head halter traction should not place the cervical spine in extension except by specific directions from the physician. The neck is maintained in neutral or slight flexion by the directional pull of the pulley system from the spreader bar. More pressure should be be applied to the occipital piece of the head halter than to the chin piece.

The traction is applied with the patient supine or sitting in bed (Fig. 14-3). The desired position of the patient's trunk determines the directional pull and placement of the pulley system. Frequently both positions are utilized by changing between two pulley systems and altering the elevation of the head of the bed.

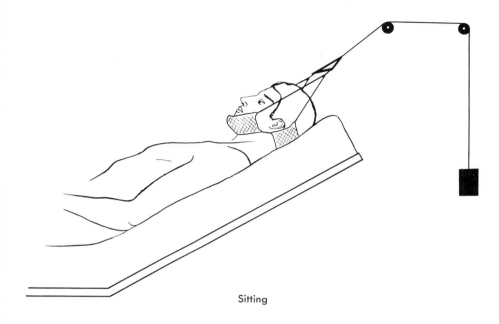

Sitting

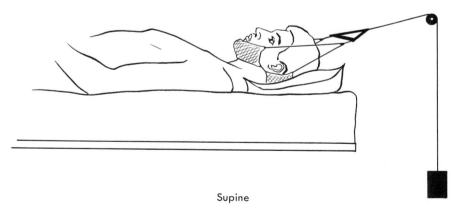

Supine

Fig. 14-3. Head halter traction—two positions.

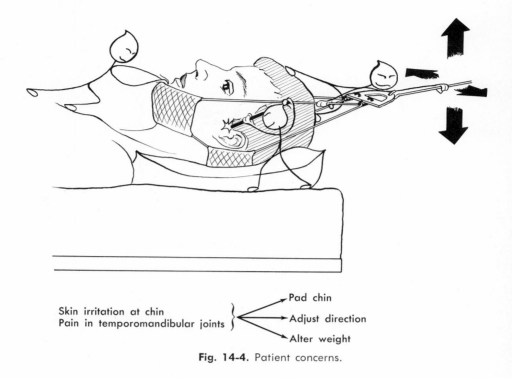

Skin irritation at chin
Pain in temporomandibular joints ⟩ ⟵ Pad chin
Adjust direction
Alter weight

Fig. 14-4. Patient concerns.

Regardless of the patient's position, he must be comfortable and the apparatus functioning properly.

CHECKING THE PATIENT. After the application of the apparatus, the patient should be asked for any specific complaints. A slight adjustment of the head halter or pulley system frequently averts the necessity of a second trip. When subsequent visits or patient rounds are made, the patient's two most frequent complaints are pain in the temporomandibular joints and irritation of the skin under the chin (Fig. 14-4). The discomfort in the temporomandibular joint is caused by upward pressure on the undersurface of the jaw and may be relieved by altering the direction of the pulley system and increasing the pressure on the occipital pad or by decreasing the weight. The skin of the chin should be checked prior to attempts to relieve the irritation. The latter may be accomplished by decreasing the weight or appropriately padding the chin piece. Minor complaints are usually resolved by minimal adjustment in the apparatus. If the patient's complaints continue, despite multiple alterations, the traction should be removed and the physician advised.

CHECKING THE APPARATUS. The head halter must fit comfortably without localized pressure. The pulley system must direct the traction force in the correct line and be operational, that is, the knots secure, the rope gliding freely in the pulleys, and the weights hanging free.

PELVIC TRACTION

INDICATIONS. Pelvic traction is applied to the lumbar spine by a belt applied just above and surrounding the iliac crests. This treatment is used primarily for acute or chronic low back pain with or without sciatica. The traction may be beneficial in the management of the acute back sprain, herniated nucleus pulposus, and degenerative arthritis of the lumbar spine. These conditions have some overlap and are probably all related to problems in the intervertebral disk.

The most important accomplishment of pelvic traction is to keep a patient recumbent and relatively quiet. When a patient enters the hospital for "traction," this event suggests that the back will somehow be stretched and the disks "popped" into place. This is not the case. The 20 to 30 pounds of traction applied to the pelvis is dissipated primarily by friction of the belt on the skin and the buttocks and thighs on the bed. Although the apparatus does not provide significant intervertebral disk distraction, the enforced bed rest is beneficial.

APPARATUS AND APPLICATION. Pelvic traction is applied using a pelvic belt, spreader bar, and pulley system. The patient is positioned supine on the open belt with the top edge of the latter approximately 2 inches above the iliac crests. The device is fastened snugly in front over the lower abdomen to gain a purchase on the crests. Proper fitting is difficult on the obese patient, for if the belt is tight enough to grip the pelvis, the abdomen may be uncomfortably compressed. If the device is too loose, it will slide off the crests and not afford any purchase. A pelvic band that maintains its position fairly well (Fig. 14-5) is usually found by trial and error with an assortment of sizes.

The pelvic belt has two lateral tapes at the bottom edge that extend 3 or 4 feet. These tapes are held apart by and connect to a spreader bar that connects to the pulley system. From 20 to 30 pounds is recommended to ensure the patient the sensation of "traction" and to keep the belt from pulling loose or causing skin irritation. The traction force is applied gradually and not with a sudden jerk.

POSITION. The direction of the traction does not determine the amount of flexion or extension of the lumbar spine. Adjustment of the bed positions the spine in the desired attitude. Semi-Fowler's position with the head of the bed elevated 18 to 20 inches, the hips flexed 35 to 40 degrees, and the legs parallel to the floor is recommended. The buttocks lie in a valley in the bed, preventing the patient from being pulled to the foot, and the legs are elevated, decreasing the risk of thromboembolic complications. This position is usually comfortable and, by flexing the lumbar

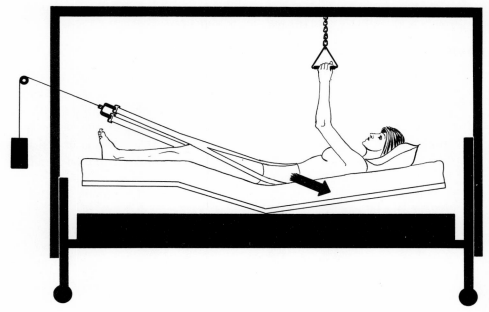

Fig. 14-5. Pelvic traction.

spine, increases the size of the intervertebral foramina. The pulley system is directed in line with or slightly below the long axis of the thighs.

CHECKING THE PATIENT. The patient should be asked initially and when making subsequent rounds about the fit of the belt. This is the most frequent complaint and often requires multiple changes. The patient sometimes slides down from the pull and his feet rest on the edge of the bed. This may be corrected by lowering the head of the bed or elevating the foot. Other complaints referable to apparatus can usually be resolved by changing the position of the bed, altering the direction of pull, or varying the amount of weight. If the patient complains of increased back or leg pain in traction, the pelvic belt should be removed and the physician notified.

CHECKING THE APPARATUS. The pelvic belt must fit snugly and its lateral tapes be free of the thighs and attached securely to the spreader bar. The pulley system must be operational and properly directing the traction force.

TEMPORARY ANKLE TRACTION

INDICATIONS. A fractured femur cannot be adequately splinted without traction to overcome associated muscle spasm. Temporary partial immobilization is afforded by circumferential traction applied to the ankle with the limb supported in a Thomas splint. Countertraction is provided

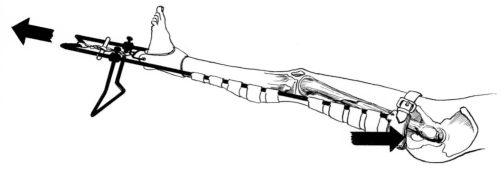

Fig. 14-6. Temporary ankle traction for femoral fracture.

by pressure of the splint against the ischial tuberosity. The apparatus is useful in the transfer of the injured patient prior to definitive treatment.

APPARATUS AND APPLICATION. A Thomas splint is prepared with slings to support the thigh and leg. Gentle traction is manually applied to the foot and the malleoli padded. With the entire limb supported and the traction maintained, the ring of the Thomas splint is placed against the ischial tuberosity. The lower extremity is gently lowered into the splint and, with traction still maintained, the ankle gripped with either a figure-eight cloth or the special ankle harness. The encircling device is attached under tension to the end of the splint. The traction may be increased by the use of a stick between the sides of the splint acting as a Spanish windlass. The entire lower extremity is wrapped to the splint from ankle to groin for additional security (Fig. 14-6).

PRECAUTIONS. This type of traction should never be in place for more than 3 or 4 hours. Pressure necrosis of skin about the ankle develops rapidly. If immobilization is necessary for a longer period, the traction must be released for 15 minutes and then reapplied.

CHAPTER 15

SKIN TRACTION

DEFINITION

Skin traction utilizes the friction between tapes and the skin to exert a directional force. Skin tapes are placed lengthwise on opposite sides of an extremity and held snugly in position by an encircling wrap. The force is applied to the limb by pulling on the free ends of the tapes, and it cannot exceed the tolerance of skin to traction or the friction between the surfaces. Skin traction is restricted to the extremities and can only apply 5 to 7 pounds of longitudinal force safely. This type of traction does not adequately control rotation. To prevent skin breakdown, the duration of continuous traction should not exceed 3 to 4 weeks.

INDICATIONS

Skin traction is most valuable in the management of specific children's fractures. These injuries do not require large forces for alignment or immobilization, and the gentle pull of skin traction is sufficient and safe. The skin tolerates the traction well for the short time needed for fracture healing.

Fractures in adults are difficult to treat in skin traction. The forces required to reduce and maintain alignment frequently exceed the tolerance of skin. Rotational deformity cannot be satisfactorily controlled and the prolonged time required for adult fracture healing makes continuous skin traction hazardous. The adult fractures usually treated by skin traction are stable, and the skin tapes may be removed and reapplied without loss of position. The traction provides patient comfort by a gentle steadying force associated with support.

Skin traction is often applied to an adult fracture for a short period prior to definitive treatment. This action provides limited immobilization, enhances patient comfort, and temporizes the situation satisfactorily.

Skin traction is occasionally employed to steady a reduced joint dislocation. Once again the forces required are not great and are not needed for a prolonged time. The traction partially immobilizes and provides patient comfort. If the reduction is potentially unstable and re-dislocation is a concern, skin traction is usually not sufficient.

GENERAL CONSIDERATIONS
Materials

The skin tapes are either individually fashioned from moleskin or ad-hesive tape or are commercially available in a variety of materials and sizes. Regardless of type, one side of the tape adheres to the skin and is held in place by the encircling wrap. Some tapes adhere more securely and apparently permit a greater force to be applied. This is not the case, however, for skin tolerance is the limiting factor in the amount of trac-tion. The tapes are placed lengthwise on opposite sides of the limb and extend beyond the limits of the extremity. They should be as long and as wide as the specific setup permits to distribute the traction force on as much skin as possible. The ends of the tapes are fastened to a spreader bar, which directs the traction in line with each tape and attaches to the pulley system. An Ace bandage holds the tapes snugly against the limb.

Skin

The tapes should not be placed on skin that is abraded or that has a superficial infection or rash. Covering skin with these conditions increases the risk of skin breakdown and other complications.

Excessive hair is rarely a problem in children; however, shaving may be necessary in the adult. Skin preparation prior to application of the skin tapes varies. The skin must be clean and dry, but wiping off with ether is usually not necessary. A liquid adhesive may be beneficial, though the skin tapes usually adhere satisfactorily without it. Commercial tapes frequently are accompanied by instruction pertaining to skin care for the specific product.

Bony prominences

Skin tapes should not be placed over the bony prominences. The skin in these areas does not tolerate the traction force and rapidly breaks down. The bony prominences should be protected with cotton padding of the type used with plaster of Paris.

Application

The skin tapes are positioned with the limb supported and gentle traction being applied. The tapes must extend far enough beyond the extremity for attachment of the spreader bar. The opposing tapes do not surround the limb completely, and an exposed strip of skin is left on either side. The tapes are then applied to the skin and held by an Ace

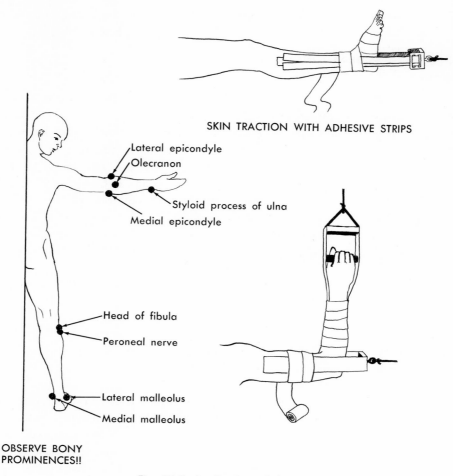

SKIN TRACTION WITH ADHESIVE STRIPS

Lateral epicondyle
Olecranon
Styloid process of ulna
Medial epicondyle

Head of fibula
Peroneal nerve

Lateral malleolus
Medial malleolus

OBSERVE BONY
PROMINENCES!!

Fig. 15-1. Application of skin traction.

bandage wrap. The wrap is from distal to proximal and is snug but not constrictive. The free tape ends are attached to the spreader bar and thus the pulley system. The limb continues to be supported until the traction force is gradually applied by the previously positioned pulley system (Fig. 15-1).

A line is drawn on the skin immediately adjacent to the proximal ends of the tapes. This marker readily establishes any slippage of the tapes.

Support

The limb in skin traction must have adequate support. This should be attended to simultaneously with application.

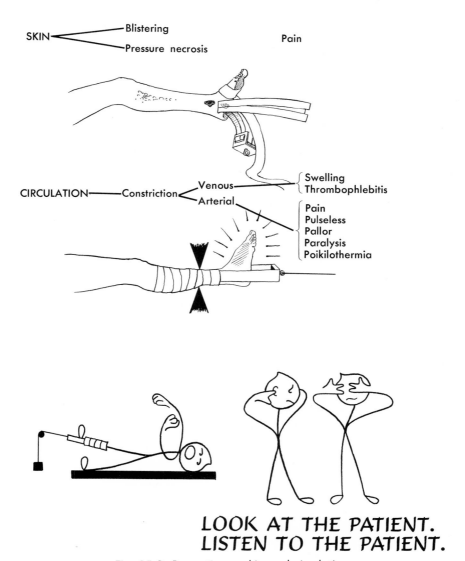

SKIN — Blistering
— Pressure necrosis

Pain

CIRCULATION — Constriction — Venous — Swelling
Thrombophlebitis

Arterial — Pain
Pulseless
Pallor
Paralysis
Poikilothermia

LOOK AT THE PATIENT.
LISTEN TO THE PATIENT.

Fig. 15-2. Precautions—skin and circulation.

Countertraction

The type of traction, size of the patient, and weight applied will determine whether a specific countertraction force is necessary. This is evaluated at the time of application and, if required, is accomplished by tilting the bed appropriately and using the patient's body weight.

Precautions

SKIN. The most frequent complication of this form of traction is skin necrosis. The shearing force of the tape causes blistering and then full thickness skin loss. These lesions are prevented by careful padding prior to tape application and limiting the amount of weight used. Slippage of the tapes is often accompanied by skin damage. The skin must be thoroughly checked if it occurs.

If skin necrosis or blistering develops, skin traction may not be reapplied to the area. The injury also prevents pin insertion or surgery locally because of the risk of infection. For these reasons skin tapes should not be placed over areas in which subsequent surgery or pin insertion is contemplated. The pressure from the tapes may also cause nerve injuries. Superficial nerves must be protected by appropriate padding (Fig. 15-2).

CIRCULATION. The venous and arterial circulation may be compromised by the constriction of a tightly wrapped Ace bandage or the twisting of a limb in the apparatus. The symptoms and signs have been described in Chapter 9 and are the same. The skin traction must be removed if there is a suspicion of circulatory embarrassment. Failure to do so will create serious problems.

TYPES OF TRACTION
Dunlop's traction

INDICATIONS. Supracondylar fractures in children with posterior displacement of the distal fragment and marked swelling of the antecubital fossa are satisfactorily treated by Dunlop's traction.

DESCRIPTION. The traction is applied with the patient supine and his trunk flush with the edge of the bed. The affected extremity is supported and placed in 90 degrees of abduction off the side of the bed. The bony prominences of the wrist are protected and skin tapes applied to the supinated forearm with the elbow extended. While support is maintained, a sling is placed over the arm just proximal to the elbow to permit a traction force toward the floor, and the skin tapes are fastened to the spreader bar, which attaches to the pulley system. Weights are gradually added to the sling and the pulley system until the elbow maintains a position of 45 degrees of flexion. The vectors of force in line with the forearm and perpendicular to the arm create a resultant force along the axis of the humerus. This combined force reduces and maintains fracture alignment. From

4 to 5 pounds is usually required for the forearm and 1 to 2 pounds for the arm. Dunlop's is one of the few skin tractions that does not support or cradle the limb. The light weight of the child's upper extremity may be safely held by the skin tapes. A heavier arm could not be controlled in this manner (Fig. 15-3).

COUNTERTRACTION. Specific measures to apply countertraction are usually not necessary, for the forces involved are insufficient. If needed, the edge of the bed may be raised and the body weight used.

SPECIAL CONSIDERATIONS. Supracondylar fractures may be associated with circulatory embarrassment, and the latter is increased by elbow flexion.

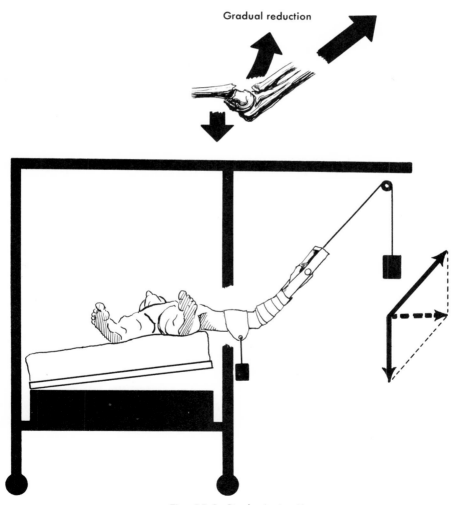

Gradual reduction

Fig. 15-3. Dunlop's traction.

Dunlop's traction permits reduction of the fracture with the elbow in partial extension and lessens the risk from compression in the antecubital fossa.

Bryant's traction

INDICATIONS. The fractured femur in the infant weighing 40 pounds or less is difficult to manage by conventional traction apparatus, because the lower extremities are short and the perineum must be exposed for diaper changes. Bryant's traction is suitable for treatment of this injury. It applies a gentle force in line with the femur but does not interfere with personal hygiene. This setup is also useful in the closed reduction of a congenital dislocation of the hip by gentle traction with increasing abduction to the hips.

This form of treatment is not recommended for children above the weight of 40 pounds. With each additional pound, the risks of skin traction increase.

DESCRIPTION. The patient is supine with a restraining strap at least 6 inches wide placed across the abdomen. Both lower extremities are flexed at the hips to 90 degrees and supported with the knees extended by the feet. With the patient held in this position, the region of the malleoli and fibular head is padded and skin tapes are applied to both the injured and the uninjured extremities. The tapes extend 2 to 3 inches above the knee joint and are held with Ace bandage wraps. The spreader bars are attached and the patient's position is maintained by two pulley systems.

The pulley systems should exert a force that *just does not* lift the buttocks off the bed. This is sufficient to maintain adequate length and alignment. The force required is in the order of 1 to 2 pounds, and rarely 3. If the weight applied *just* raises the buttocks off the bed, the child may increase this distance by his wiggling and suspend his lower trunk by his legs. This places too much tension on the skin through the tapes. Counteraction is automatically provided by the patient's body (Fig. 15-4).

Both legs must be placed in traction to prevent the patient from rotating around one extremity. This might cause not only a rotational malunion at the fracture site but circulatory embarrassment from the torsion.

This type of traction with minor modifications is suitable for the closed reduction of an infant's congenital dislocation of the hip. The child lies transversely in the bed and the lower extremities are placed in skin traction through two attached pulley systems. Progressive abduction of the hips is accomplished by gradually spreading the two pulley systems. The weights involved are comparable to those used in the management of an infant's femur.

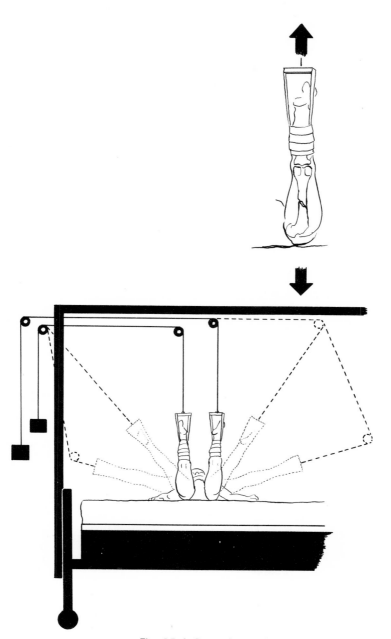

Fig. 15-4. Bryant's traction.

SPECIAL CONSIDERATIONS. The infant does not offer verbal complaints, so any change in his apparent comfort must be carefully evaluated. The patient's position, traction apparatus, and pulley system should be inspected for untoward changes at least daily. The most serious complication of this traction is circulatory embarrassment. This may be caused not only by constriction of the Ace wrap but also by twisting of a leg with the child's movements. Both the injured and the uninjured sides have been damaged by this complication, and frequent checks of the circulation in both feet are mandatory.

Russell's skin traction

INDICATIONS. Fractures of the femoral shaft in children weighing from 40 to 80 pounds are adequately aligned and immobilized with Russell's skin traction.

DESCRIPTION. This traction applies two vectors of force to the distal femur and aligns and maintains length at the fracture site. One force is applied to the back of the thigh and brings the distal femur anteriorly, while the other is applied in the long axis of the leg. The traction apparatus may have a single pulley system (single Russell's) or a double system (split Russell's).

The apparatus is applied with the patient supine and the affected leg supported in gentle traction. A sling is slipped under the distal thigh and attached to a spreader bar. Skin tapes with proper padding, Ace bandage, and spreader bar are applied to the leg. The traction forces are then gradually applied either through two pulley systems or by a single system with the weights at the end of the bed. The forces result in some flexion of the hip and knee. The leg should remain parallel to the floor, supported by pillows. The amount of traction required on the leg is approximately double that on the thigh and is in the order of 6 and 3 pounds, respectively, depending on the size of the child. The three distal pulleys in single Russell's traction conveniently double the force of the distal weight on the leg; however, pull on the sling is not changed (Fig. 15-5).

The countertraction of the patient's body weight may be increased by elevation of the foot of the bed.

SPECIAL CONSIDERATIONS. The magnitude and the direction of the resultant of the two force vectors can be altered by changing the amounts of weight applied and the line of traction from the thigh sling. The apparatus permits alignment of the distal to the proximal fragment. Adequate reduction is determined by serial x-rays. The usual precautions with skin traction should be observed, including monitoring of the patient and apparatus.

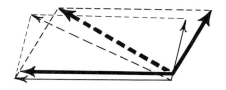

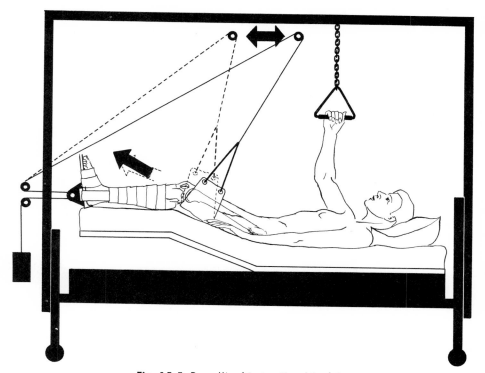

Fig. 15-5. Russell's skin traction (single).

Buck's extension skin traction

INDICATIONS. Unilateral Buck's traction may be used for temporary immobilization of a fractured hip prior to definitive therapy. This treatment does not attempt reduction but steadies the extremity in the position of deformity for patient comfort. If surgery is delayed beyond 3 or 4 days, the skin traction should be replaced by skeletal traction. Bilateral Buck's skin traction is indicated with some pain syndromes of the low back. As with pelvic traction, the distraction force is negligible; however, the patient is kept recumbent and quiet. This form of traction is occasionally used to partially immobilize stable injuries of the knee or proximal tibia.

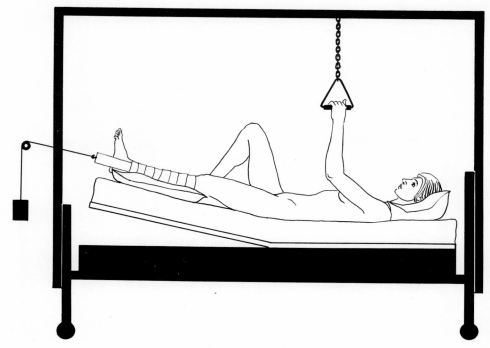

Fig. 15-6. Buck's extension traction.

DESCRIPTION. Buck's extension skin traction is applied by tapes held to the leg by a wrap after padding the proximal fibula and both malleoli. The spreader bar joins the pulley system of the end of the bed. The amount of traction should not exceed 5 to 7 pounds (Fig. 15-6).

If the traction is used on a fractured hip, the lower extremity should be cradled with pillows for additional support.

The patient with bilateral Buck's traction for low back pain is usually most comfortable with the bed in semi-Fowler's position. This attitude flexes the lumbar spine and opens the intervertebral foramina. Semi-Fowler's position also stabilizes the buttocks in a valley of the bed and keeps the legs elevated.

SPECIAL CONSIDERATIONS. Particular attention must be given the areas of the fibular head and malleoli. A peroneal palsy that develops during treatment of a benign low back syndrome is an unwarranted complication. A pressure sore from skin tapes used to temporarily immobilize a fractured hip may take longer to heal than the bone injury.

CHAPTER 16

SKELETAL TRACTION

general considerations

DEFINITION

Skeletal traction applies force directly to bone by means of metallic devices placed in the osseous tissue. The traction forces may exert 20 to 30 pounds of pull and be maintained for 3 to 4 months without ill effect.

The magnitude of skeletal traction frequently requires specific measures for countertraction in addition to the patient's body weight. The increased countertraction is usually provided by appropriate elevation of the ends or side of the bed.

Skeletal traction applies not only longitudinal pull to a bone but permits control of rotation. This factor is important in fracture alignment (Fig. 16-1).

The management of a fracture just begins with the application of the apparatus. A patient "in traction" requires continuous observation of patient and equipment, numerous major and minor adjustments, and multiple followup x-rays. The judgments and skills demanded by this form of treatment

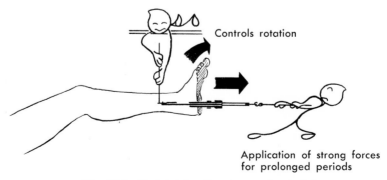

Controls rotation

Application of strong forces
for prolonged periods

Fig. 16-1. Skeletal traction: general principles.

are just as critical as for an open reduction. The proper use of skeletal traction is a meticulous art.

INDICATIONS

Skeletal traction is an excellent method to reduce certain fractures, maintain their alignment, and provide limited immobilization. Although it is most often employed in adults, skeletal traction is indicated in specific children's fractures.

Fractures in bones surrounded by a large muscle mass, such as the femur, shorten and angulate secondary to muscle spasm. Skeletal traction permits this fracture to be held out to length, despite strong muscular forces. Markedly comminuted fractures of the major long bones with significant overriding are frequently placed in skeletal traction to prevent shortening. Unstable fractures of the long bones, which easily displace in plaster, may be maintained in satisfactory alignment by skeletal traction. Displaced fractures of the pelvis frequently are reduced and maintained with this form of treatment. Skeletal traction employing skull tongs is the only satisfactory method of applying controlled forces to unstable injuries of the cervical spine. Other methods may permanently injure the spinal cord.

Reduced unstable dislocations and fracture-dislocations are often held in position by skeletal traction until healing occurs. The direction and magnitude of the force prevent redisplacement of the injury.

The injury must not only be suitable, but the patient's general condition must be satisfactory to employ skeletal traction. This method of treatment requires a prolonged period of recumbency that the patient may not be able to tolerate. All the variables must be evaluated prior to the decision to use skeletal traction.

MATERIALS AND EQUIPMENT

The insertion of metallic devices into bone and the application of skeletal traction require a variety of paraphernalia. These materials and equipment must be available, organized, and set up prior to working directly with the patient. Everything should be ready to go, for delays increase patient anxiety and discomfort. A foreknowledge of the type of traction to be applied will dictate the specifics, but all forms have common denominators.

Kirschner wires, Steinmann pins, and traction bows

A long list of metallic devices to apply traction to bone is available. With the exception of skull tongs for cervical spine traction, however, the Kirschner wire and the Steinmann pin are sufficient and adaptable for most conditions. Kirschner wires and Steinmann pins are round stainless steel rods with a point at one or both ends. Both are available with a smooth or threaded surface and with a trocar or diamond point. The two differ in size. The diameter of a Kirschner wire ranges from 0.035 to 0.0625 inch, while that of a Steinmann pin varies from $\frac{5}{64}$ to $\frac{3}{16}$ inch.

Both pins are usually inserted perpendicular to and completely through the bone. The traction force is applied to the wire or pin by the appropriate traction bow.

The traction bows should not impinge on skin. If the bow is too small or the traction improperly conceived, pressure between the device and skin may result. This situation is readily avoided (Fig. 16-2).

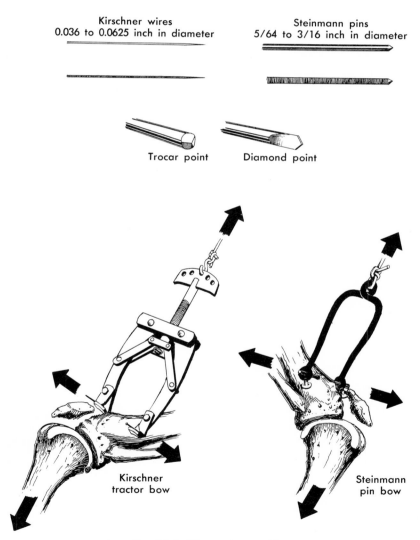

Kirschner wires
0.036 to 0.0625 inch in diameter

Steinmann pins
5/64 to 3/16 inch in diameter

Trocar point   Diamond point

Kirschner
tractor bow

Steinmann
pin bow

Fig. 16-2. Wires, pins, and bows.

The Steinmann pin traction bow attaches to both ends of the pin but applies no longitudinal traction on it. The pin is strong enough to transmit considerable force without bending.

The Kirschner wire tractor bow grips and exerts longitudinal traction to the wire. The ends are fixed in the tractor bow between a toothed device and a flat surface, and, by spreading the bow, tension is applied to the wire. This tension prevents the slim wire from bending when a perpendicular force is exerted by the bow.

The Kirschner wire makes a much smaller hole in skin and bone than the Steinmann pin and, on this basis, may have some advantages. This theoretically might decrease the risk of infection, damage to bone, and injury to vital structures.

Skull tongs

Skull tongs are necessary to apply skeletal traction to the head. There are several types, namely the Crutchfield, Barton, and Vincke. However, they all gain their purchase on the skull by penetrating the outer table without violating the inner table. The tongs are attached to a pulley system for traction.

Hand drill, chuck key, and pin cutter

Both the Kirschner wire and Steinmann pins are inserted with a hand drill. Placement of skull tongs requires not only the drill but drill bits of the correct size to make the initial hole in the outer table. The chuck key ensures that the wire, pin, or bit is held tightly in the drill during use. Any excess pin or wire is removed after insertion with the pin cutter.

Pulley system

The pulley system has been described and, for the purpose of this discussion, includes the rope, pulleys, weight carries, and weights as well as the magnitude and alignment of the specific traction force. No attempt shall be made to describe placement of specific pulleys, crossbars, or weights. These are left to the operator's ingenuity with the equipment at hand.

Bed and fracture frame

Skeletal traction requires a fixed pulley system and thus is applied with the patient in bed or on a special fracture frame. The bed does not need to be electrical, with switches to raise and lower various parts as well as the entire bed. Such invention may be inadvisable, for an inadvertent touch of a switch can throw the traction out of alignment. The hospital bed with a firm mattress that independently elevates the head and foot and that accepts a fracture frame is sufficient. Tilting the entire bed lengthwise or from side to side is accomplished satisfactorily with shock blocks.

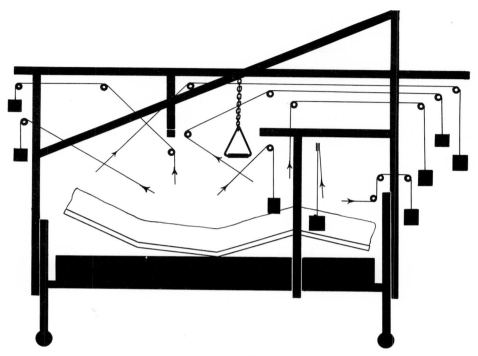

Fig. 16-3. "Erector set."

Special apparatus such as the Foster or Stryker frame and the CircO-lectric bed facilitate nursing of the patient in skeletal cervical spine traction with or without paraplegia.

The fracture frame and attached cross, extension, and side bars permit placement of the pulleys in specific locations to direct the traction forces. After the overhead frame is secured, the parts are joined like an erector set to accomplish this purpose. The various bars must be in the correct positions for the pulley systems and securely joined together. If the "erector set" is stable and performs its function, the type and setup of the apparatus are secondary (Fig. 16-3).

The fracture frame, "erector set," and usually a trapeze are set up before handling the patient. There may be minor adjustments after the patient is "in traction"; however, to facilitate care the apparatus must already be functional.

Special equipment

The type of skeletal traction determines the need for special materials and equipment. Slings, tubular stockinette, and foot plates are made available as needed. The Thomas splint, Pearson attachment, and Böhler-

Braun frame will be described in relation with their use for specific types of traction (see Chapter 17).

PIN INSERTICN
General considerations

The site of pin insertion determines the exact location to which the traction force is applied. The position is determined by the specific injury and the apparatus to be employed. The decision also requires evaluation of overall treatment plan and pertinent local factors.

SKIN. The area of proposed pin insertion must be free of superficial infection, abrasions, or rashes. The placement of a pin through these conditions risks a pin tract infection that may completely defeat the treatment plan. The insertion of a skeletal pin creates an "open fracture" with the hazard of osteomyelitis.

The skeletal device must not be placed near the possible site of a subsequent surgical procedure. Despite adequate precaution, low-grade infection is common at the pin tract and prevents operative intervention in this area while the wound is open.

MUSCLE AND TENDON. The pin ideally should pass only through skin, subcutaneous tissue, and bone. Occasionally the device must course through muscle and tendon; however, this should be avoided if possible.

ARTERY AND NERVE. The placement of skeletal pins requires knowledge of the specific anatomic location of vital structures. Permanent residual disability may result from penetration of an artery or a nerve by careless insertion and exceed that from the original injury. The neurovascular status of the part must be determined before pin insertion, and after the traction has been applied it must be carefully monitored.

JOINTS. Traction pins should not penetrate joints. The potential complication of a pyarthrosis is too great a risk. The traction force should avoid pulling across a joint. The prolonged stretching of the structures around a joint results in a chronic strain with potential joint stiffness. Frequently this consideration in placement must be compromised for anatomic reasons. Skeletal traction on a hemipelvis should usually be exerted through the ipsilateral femur and through the hip joint. Traction to the femur, however, often requires the skeletal pin to be placed in the proximal tibia.

BONE. The traction pins are best placed in the metaphysis just proximal or distal to the open or closed epiphyseal line. Pins should avoid the epiphysis, because of the closeness to the joint, and the diaphysis, to prevent significant loss of strength associated with a predisposition to pathologic fracture. Pins crossing or near the epiphyseal plate can retard growth and cause resultant deformity and shortening. The growth plate must not be penetrated.

The fracture hematoma must not be violated by the skeletal pins. This

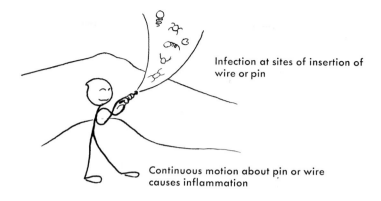

Infection at sites of insertion of
wire or pin

Continuous motion about pin or wire
causes inflammation

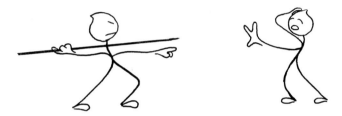

Impinging or penetrating vital structures with
wire or pin (nerves, arteries, joints,
and epiphyseal plates)

Fig. 16-4. Hazards of pin insertion.

infraction converts a closed fracture to an open fracture with the potential adverse sequelae (Fig. 16-4).

Procedure

CONSENT. The insertion of a pin in bone is a surgical procedure and requires a signed consent form from the patient to proceed. The patient should be advised of the necessity of the surgery and steps that will be followed. The procedure requires either local or general anesthesia, and the type must be indicated on the consent slip.

SETUP. The placement of a metallic device in bone creates an open fracture. Strict surgical asepsis must be followed to minimize pin tract infections. The latter are difficult to eradicate and usually upset the management plan.

All the materials must be sterile with the exception of the traction bow. The drill, chuck key, pins and wires, scalpel and blades, and drapes are all laid out on a sterile field. Syringes, needles, local anesthetic, and sponges are also available. The fracture bed is already prepared with the "erector set" and pulleys to attach the pin to the pulley system.

STABILIZING THE LIMB. Regardless of whether the patient is on a bed, gurney, or operating room table, the limb in the area of the pin insertion must be supported and steadied. The stabilization is often accompanied by gentle traction.

SKIN PREPARATION. The approximate locations of the skin entrance and exit wounds are identified, shaved, and given a routine surgical preparation. The latter must be thorough to prevent an osteomyelitis and its possible sequelae.

TECHNIQUE. The operator performs a routine surgical scrub and applies sterile gloves. The remainder of the procedure is carried out using aseptic techniques. The sites of entrance and exit are identified and sterilely draped.

If local anesthesia is to be used, the patient should be specifically asked about allergies to such drugs prior to administration. If there is no allergy, the site of entrance and anticipated exit are infiltrated with 1% to 2% procaine or lidocaine superficially and then down to bone. This type of anesthesia is usually satisfactory, particularly if complimented by parenteral analgesia.

The appropriately sized wire or pin is placed and tightened in the drill with approximately 2 inches exposed. If additional pin or wire is out of the drill, the former is difficult to direct and bends on contact with the bone.

A stab wound is made with a scalpel at the previously anesthetized entrance site, and the pin is pushed directly to the bone. The bone is reached when the point of the pin hits a firm resistance. Care should be exercised at this point to align the wire perpendicular to the longitudinal axis of the bone. The pin or wire is drilled through bone using minimal force, having the trocar or diamond point cut its own course with multiple turns. The penetration of the pin through each cortex is associated with a definite "giving" sensation that must be appreciated to ensure placement of the pin in the bone. As the pin is drilled out the opposite side of the bone, more local anesthesia may be required. When the pin tents on exiting, a small incision is made over the tip to prevent twisting the skin. The pin is drilled through a sufficient length to permit application of the traction bow. The drill is removed and dry or moist sterile dressings are applied around the end of the pin and secured with bias-cut stockinette. Either a Steinmann pin bow or a Kirschner tractor bow is applied and the excess pin or wire removed. The sharp ends of both should be covered to prevent scratching patient, personnel, and linens. The patient is now ready to be placed "in traction."

Sites of insertion *(Fig. 16-5)*

SKULL. Each side of the skull tongs penetrates and grips the outer table of the skull above and slightly behind the external auditory meatus. The exact location varies with the type of tong; however, they all have their

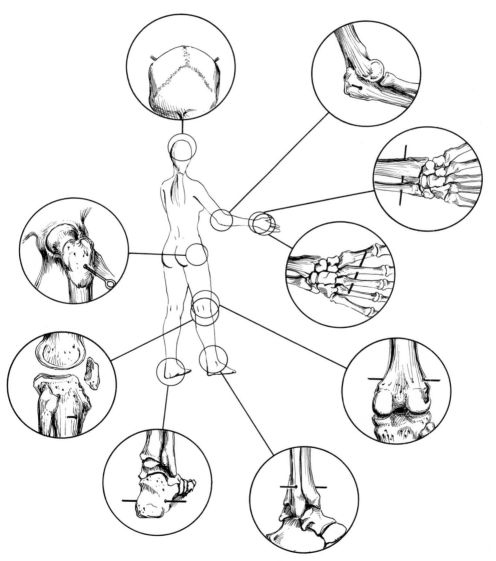

Fig. 16-5. Points of insertion.

special drills to prevent penetration of the inner table. The tongs are attached to the pulley system and must be monitored for signs of infection.

PROXIMAL ULNA. The pin is placed 1 inch distal to the tip of olecranon process and ¼ to ⅜ inch anterior to the subcutaneous proximal ulna. The pin should penetrate both ulnar cortices but not be deep enough to injure any neurovascular structures. The olecranon pin is inserted from the medial to lateral forearm after careful palpation of the ulnar nerve. This method of insertion prevents skewering the nerve with possible permanent residual disability.

DISTAL FEMUR. The distal femoral pin is inserted 1 to 2 inches proximal to the adductor tubercle and approximately ½ inch anterior to this bony prominence. This location avoids injury to the major neurovascular structures as they leave the medial posterior thigh and enter the popliteal fossa. If the pin is placed more anteriorly, the femur may be missed and the suprapatellar expansion of the knee joint penetrated. Pin insertion should be from the medial to lateral thigh to protect the vital structures. The traction hoop must clear the flexed knee and not cause pressure on the anterior proximal leg.

PROXIMAL TIBIA. The proximal tibial pin is placed perpendicular to the long axis of the tibia 1 inch distal and ½ inch posterior to the tibial tubercle. After careful palpation of the peroneal nerve, insertion is from lateral to medial to avoid this structure.

DISTAL TIBIA. The pin or wire for distal tibial traction should be inserted 1½ to 2 inches proximal to the tip of the medial malleolus, perpendicular to the tibial shaft, and in the frontal plane. This location avoids entering the ankle joint. A pin or wire engaging both cortices of the tibia is adequate and may pass in front of the fibula without penetrating the latter. The direction of insertion is from medial to lateral. The traction bow applied to the pin must be sufficiently wide and not impinge the leg, and it must also be long enough to surround the sole of the foot without pressure. Frequently the foot will drop into equinus, and then pressure on the sole must be relieved by a foot plate or padding.

CALCANEUS. Calcaneal traction is applied through a pin placed 1 inch proximal and anterior to the point of the heel. After careful palpation of the posterior tibial artery, the pin is inserted from medial to lateral and perpendicular to the axis of the leg.

CHAPTER 17

SKELETAL TRACTION

anatomic considerations

SHOULDER AND ARM

Skeletal traction applied to the shoulder girdle and humerus invariably utilizes an olecranon pin. The distal humerus above the elbow joint is very thin in its anteroposterior dimension, and thus placement of the pin in the frontal plane is difficult. This location also requires the metallic device to pass through a considerable amount of soft tissues and to be uncomfortably close to vital structures. For these reasons the traction force is applied distal to and through the elbow joint.

Indications

Skeletal traction is used to treat fractures and fracture-dislocations of the shoulder girdle and fractures of the proximal, middle, and distal humerus.

Olecranon pin traction

DESCRIPTION. The patient is supine with skeletal traction applied along the axis of the humerus through an olecranon pin. The arm is maintained in one of two positions, depending on the adequacy of fracture reduction.

Position I: to the side. The arm is in 40 to 90 degrees of abduction and is supported by the bed in neutral flexion or extension. The pulley system extends off the bed at the elbow, and specific countertraction is applied by raising this side of the bed. The forearm is controlled by skin traction sufficient to maintain the weight of the arm in the desired elbow flexion with an additional pulley system (Fig. 17-1).

Position II: overhead. The olecranon pin applies traction to the arm with the shoulder abducted and flexed forward to 90 degrees through an overhead pulley system. The forearm is flexed to 90 degrees and supported by a 4- to 6-inch sling. The latter may be fixed or attached to

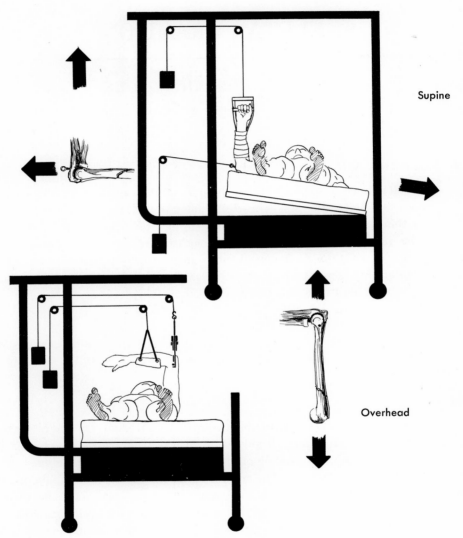

Supine

Overhead

Fig. 17-1. Olecranon pin traction.

an additional pulley system that permits active motion of the elbow. The amount of weight and exact arrangement of the pulley system are determined by the reduction.

SPECIAL CONSIDERATIONS. The traction pin must be continuously monitored for infection and for movement in the bone. Particular attention should be paid to ulnar nerve function in the hand before application of the traction and daily thereafter. Any change should be noted and promptly reported. Full thumb and finger motion are encouraged to keep the small joints limber.

HIP AND THIGH

The traction force applied to the pelvis, hip joint, or femur is usually through a pin or wire in the distal femur or the proximal tibia. In general, the skeletal pin should exert traction directly to the area of injury without transmitting the force across a joint; however, other considerations are often more important. The use of a proximal tibial pin for traction to the femoral shaft is acceptable and often preferable to a distal femoral pin. The traction setups will presume either a distal femoral or a proximal tibial pin except when specified.

Occasionally an additional force will be exerted laterally on the hip joint by skeletal pin or device in the region of the greater trochanter. This force is usually combined with a longitudinal pull for the reduction of a central fracture-dislocation of the hip.

The types of traction to the pelvis, hip, and femur differ in the amount and direction of the force applied; the position and support of the lower extremity; and the mobility of the patient and his injured part in bed. Each has its indications, advantages, and disadvantages.

Indications

Skeletal traction is used to treat fractures of the pelvis, fractures and fracture-dislocations of the acetabulum, and fractures of the proximal, middle, and distal femur.

Longitudinal traction with pillow support

DESCRIPTION. The traction is applied with the patient supine and the force exerted in line with the femur through a distal femoral or proximal tibial skeletal pin. The lower extremity is supported by pillows, usually with the hip and knee flexed and the leg horizontal with the bed. The degree of adduction or abduction is determined by the placement of the longitudinal pulley system.

The amount of traction force depends on the injury and the weight of the patient. The foot of the bed should be elevated to increase the countertraction from the patient's body weight (Fig. 17-2).

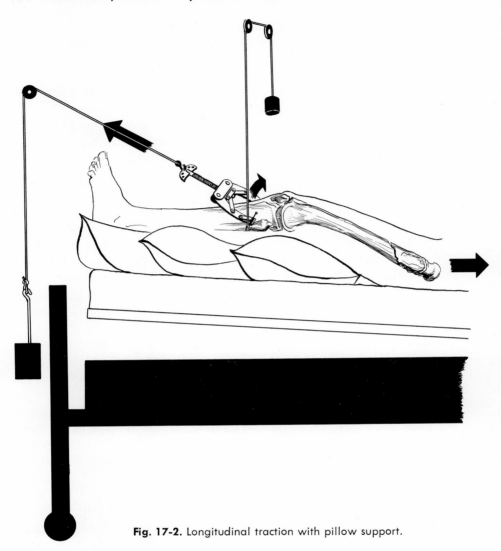

Fig. 17-2. Longitudinal traction with pillow support.

Rotation of the extremity is controlled by a separate pulley system attached to the inner or outer side of the traction bow, which is utilized for longitudinal pull. Internal or external rotational deformity can be corrected by the use of 2 to 3 pounds of force on the outer or inner aspect of the bow, respectively.

SPECIAL CONSIDERATIONS. The prime advantage of this type of traction is its simplicity and lack of apparatus. The patient's nursing needs may be readily attended to without the hindrance of apparatus. This traction is most useful in managing fractures of the intertrochanteric area of the femur.

This traction does not adequately support or align the femoral shaft or control the leg and foot. This setup does not assist the patient in active exercise of the knee and ankle.

SPECIAL PRECAUTIONS. The patient should not slide to the foot of the bed, the pulley system must not impinge on the foot, and the heel must be protected from possible pressure sores.

90-90 traction

DESCRIPTION. The patient is supine with the skeletal traction applied through a distal femoral pin. The thigh and knee are flexed to 90 degrees, with the traction force extended along the axis of the femur and perpendicular to the bed. Sufficient weight is applied to reduce the injury without distraction or lifting the patient off the bed. The leg is supported by a 6- to 8-inch sling that is either fixed or attached to a separate pulley to permit knee motion. The placement of the sling controls internal and external rotation of the distal femur. The amount of adduction and abduction is determined by the longitudinal pulley system on the femur. This type of traction does not require additional countertraction measures (Fig. 17-3).

SPECIAL CONSIDERATIONS. This type of traction is particularly useful in aligning subtrochanteric fractures in which the proximal fragment is frequently markedly flexed in an abducted position and externally rotated. The skeletal pin should be placed in the distal femur. Insertion in the proximal tibia extends the knee and does not permit support by the sling.

SPECIAL PRECAUTIONS. Considerable force is usually necessary, and special attention must be paid to the skeletal pin. Peroneal nerve function must be carefully monitored, for the region of the fibular head is vulnerable from the sling.

Longitudinal traction with a fixed Thomas splint and Pearson attachment
SPECIAL EQUIPMENT

Thomas splint. The Thomas splint was developed for the immediate splinting of humeral and femoral fractures. Its use for temporary immobilization of the fracture femur has been described. The splint is now utilized for the long-term management of femoral fractures.

The splint consists of two rods on each side of the limb joined together proximally by a ring about the part and distally by a cross bar beyond the extremity. The two metal rods converge slightly from proximal to distal to conform to the limb. After application the ring is parallel to the groin, with the lateral rod extending proximal to the area of the greater trochanter and the medial just to the perineum. This type of splint is right- or left-sided, depending on which side rod is longer.

The complete ring of the Thomas splint has been modified to a half ring

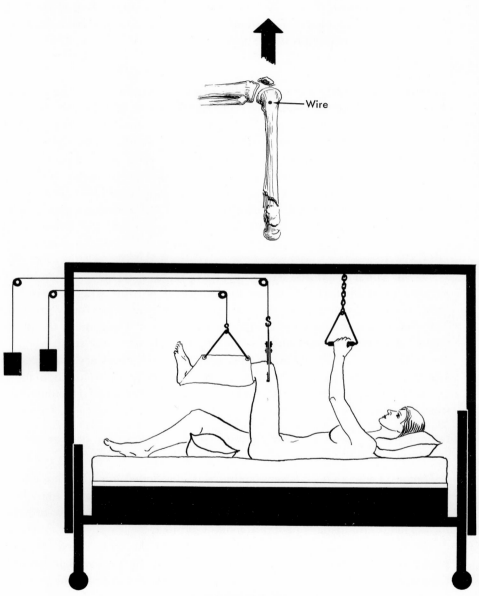

Fig. 17-3. 90-90 traction.

in the Keller-Blake splint. The latter splint may be applied with the ring either in front or in back of the proximal thigh. Placement of the ring in front of the thigh is usually recommended, with a strap posterior to it.

Prior to application of either splint, the proximal ring is padded and a continuous sling provided for support of the thigh between the two rods. The sling should be smooth and should not stretch or slide regardless of the method used.

Pearson attachment. The Pearson splint is essentially a small Thomas splint without a proximal ring. The proximal ends of the two rods have clamps that attach this splint to the rods of the Thomas splint. Hinges in the clamps permit the Pearson attachment to move independently of the larger splint. The Pearson attachment must also be provided with a smooth sling to support the leg.

The Thomas splint and Pearson attachment must be prepared and completely assembled prior to application to decrease patient discomfort.

DESCRIPTION. Longitudinal traction is applied from a distal femoral or proximal tibial pin with the patient supine. The thigh is supported by a Thomas or Keller-Blake splint, with the latter's medial proximal ring against the perineum and the distal end attached to a fixed point. The end of the splint may be attached directly to a cross bar with tape, which prevents rotation, or secured on either side with rope through a single pulley. In either case the Thomas splint is "fixed" to the bed and does not move with the patient. The ring is held against the perineum by a pulley system from the sides of proximal splint with the force directed toward the head of the bed. The half ring may be either in front or back; however, in either case it is secured to the thigh with a strap.

The leg is supported in the Pearson attachment attached to the Thomas splint at the knee joint. The end of the Pearson is either tied to the Thomas splint or joined to an independent pulley system. The former method places the knee in a fixed amount of flexion, while the latter system, if properly rigged, permits both active and passive knee motion. The patient's thigh and knee are flexed "in traction" depending on the position of the Thomas splint and the Pearson attachment. The amounts may be altered as desired by changing the fixed points or pulley systems. Thus elevating the end of the Thomas splint increases thigh flexion, and shortening the distance between the two splints decreases knee flexion. These adjustments must be coordinated with changes in the pulley system from the skeletal pin. Similarly, the amount of abduction of the lower extremity is determined both by the splints and the longitudinal traction force.

The initial placement of the Thomas splint and Pearson attachment is attempted only after the bed and "erector set" are prepared, the skeletal pin and bow are in place, and slings are fitted to the splints. The extremity is supported with gentle traction on the bow as the splints are slid gently into place. The traction is continuously maintained until transferred to the pulley system.

Increased countertraction is provided by elevation of the foot of the bed.

SPECIAL CONSIDERATIONS. The splints and pully systems require continuous monitoring. The former must maintain its relationship to the patient and the latter function without impingement. The traction is easily put out of line by general nursing care and usually needs frequent adjustments.

The apparatus is best suited for fractures in the middle or distal third of the femur, for the splints provide excellent support to the thigh. As indicated, this traction may be set up to permit either active or passive motion to the knee.

SPECIAL PRECAUTIONS. The Thomas splint must fit snugly in the perineum despite the difficulty created in using a bed pan. The adductor area should be inspected for irritation.

Rotation of the splint and leg must be prevented. A foot plate is advised if the foot tends to drop into equinus. The heel is to be protected from pressure.

The multiple ropes must not touch each other or the patient. The traction bow is not to rest on the anterior leg.

Longitudinal traction with a balanced Thomas splint and Pearson attachment (balanced suspension)

DESCRIPTION. This type of traction differs from longitudinal traction with a fixed Thomas splint only in that the latter moves with the patient as he shifts up and down in bed or lifts on the bed pan. The Thomas splint is held to the patient by balancing pulley systems from the ring and distal end. The weights at each end must be such that the splint floats or follows the extremity as the latter shifts its position. The two pulley systems may be balanced by a single weight over the patient or by separate systems. The latter is simpler, the patient need not fear the weight overhead, and the taking of portable x-rays is facilitated.

The Thomas splint and Pearson attachment are prepared and joined in a routine manner. The distal ends of the two splints are usually tied at a fixed distance, maintaining the knee in a constant amount of flexion. Precise balancing of the Thomas splint is made more difficult if there is motion between the two splints (Fig. 17-4).

The longitudinal skeletal traction is attached to a separate pulley system. The position of the lower extremity requires the coordinated adjustment of the pulley systems on the splints and the skeletal pin.

The foot of the bed is elevated to increase the amount of countertraction.

SPECIAL CONSIDERATIONS. This traction affords the patient more mobility

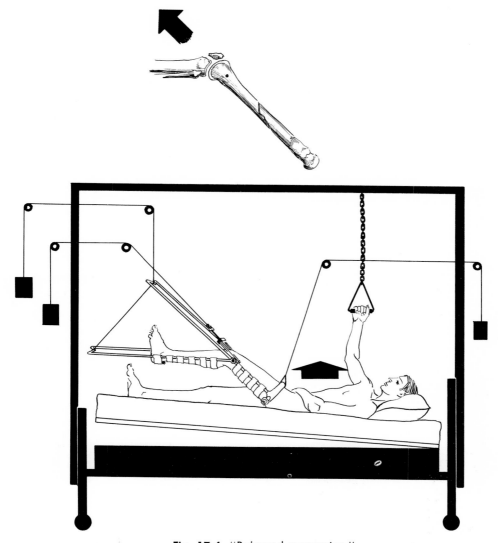

Fig. 17-4. ''Balanced suspension.''

in the apparatus. He is able to move up and down in bed and still keep a fixed relationship with the splints.

Since the pulley system is more complex, the chances of malfunction are increased. The patient and the entire system must be continuously monitored to avoid error.

SPECIAL PRECAUTIONS. Precautions are similar to those for a fixed Thomas splint, but in addition attention must be paid to the "balanced" pulley systems.

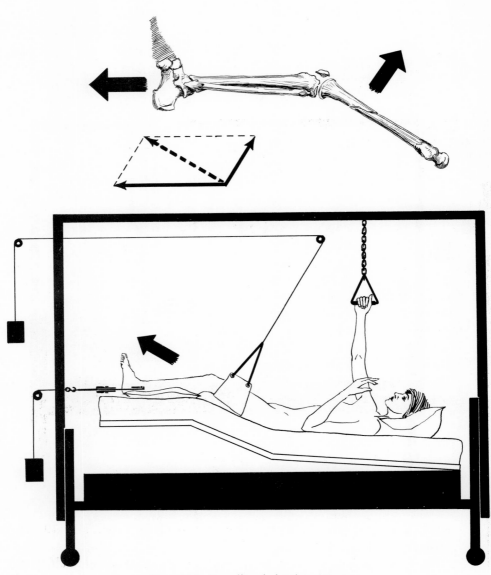

Fig. 17-5. Russell's skeletal traction.

Russell's skeletal traction

DESCRIPTION. The patient is supine and the affected lower extremity flexed moderately at the hip and knee. Skeletal traction is applied through a pin or wire in the calcaneus along the long axis of the leg. Another vector of force is applied anteriorly to the distal femur with either a pin in the distal femur or a sling behind the knee. The resultant of these two traction forces aligns and maintains reduction of the femur. The magnitude and direction of this force may be altered by changing the amount of weight or redirecting the proximal pulley system. The latter changes the sides of the parallelogram and thus the resultant.

One pulley system may apply traction to both the distal femur and the heel or two independent systems utilized (split Russell's). The leg is supported parallel with the bed and the heel protected (Fig. 17-5).

A countertraction force is frequently not necessary because of the pull on the distal femur.

SPECIAL CONSIDERATIONS. Although a sling can be used to apply force to the distal femur in conjunction with a skeletal pin in the calcaneus, skin traction should not be applied to the leg with a distal femoral pin. Skin traction cannot safely exert sufficient force on the leg to balance the skeletal pin in the femur.

This traction is simple, and the patient is not encumbered by apparatus. The peroneal area is exposed and nursing care is facilitated.

The patient should not move up or down in bed, for this will change the direction of the proximal pulley system and thus the result and force. The patient's position in bed should be noted at the time of application and maintained by frequent checks.

SPECIAL PRECAUTIONS. The thigh and leg must be supported and the heel protected. The traction requires the usual careful attention to the skeletal pins, bows, and pulley systems.

KNEE JOINT AND LEG

Skeletal traction is infrequently used to manage injuries of the knee or fractures of the tibia. Reduction and immobilization in these instances is usually satisfactorily accomplished by plaster. Occasionally, however, markedly comminuted fractures into the knee joint, markedly unstable fractures of the tibial shaft, or open fractures with associated severe soft tissue damage are best handled by skeletal traction. This type of treatment permits continuous inspection of the limb, which may be of particular value.

Longitudinal traction on the leg using a Böhler-Braun frame *(Fig. 17-6)*

SPECIAL EQUIPMENT. The Böhler-Braun frame supports the thigh and leg with the hip and knee flexed. The apparatus must be prepared with slings

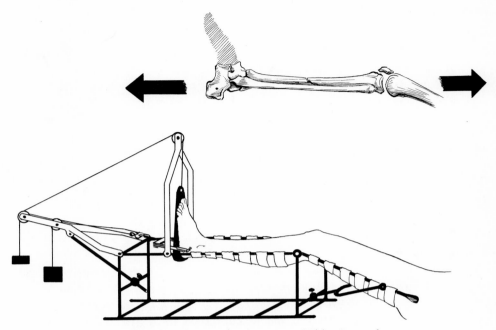

Fig. 17-6. Longitudinal traction: Böhler-Braun frame.

between metal rods similar to a Thomas splint before accepting the leg. The frame has a pulley built in for longitudinal traction on the leg as well as one to control the position of the foot.

DESCRIPTION. The patient is supine with the affected lower extremity on the Böhler-Braun frame. Skeletal traction is applied from a pin in the distal tibia or calcaneus and attached to a pulley system incorporating the frame. The foot is held in neutral position by skin tapes attached vertically to a second pulley system that is also included in the splint.

From 4 to 6 pounds of longitudinal traction is usually sufficient to overcome the muscular contraction, which is much less than that in the thigh. The alignment of the leg is controlled by the traction and the sling support.

Countertraction is afforded by the posterior flexed thigh, and raising the bed is usually not indicated.

SPECIAL CONSIDERATIONS. The primary advantages of this traction are its simplicity and the opportunity to inspect the soft tissues. The patient is also free of encumbrances with the exception of the leg, and nursing care is facilitated.

SPECIAL PRECAUTIONS. This method of treatment may distract the fracture fragments and delay or prevent union. This possible complication must be recognized and avoided.

CHAPTER 18

ORTHOPAEDIC HISTORY

A patient's orthopaedic history is an accumulation of pertinent facts that describe a particular problem and point to a specific diagnosis. The appropriate treatment may be rendered only on the basis of the correct diagnosis.

The information is best obtained by direct questioning of the patient. The rapport developed between the examiner and the patient is of the utmost importance. The latter's confidence must be gained through consideration of his privacy and personal identity. The patient has sought

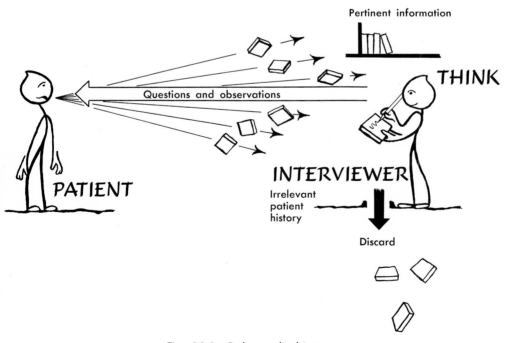

Fig. 18-1. Orthopaedic history.

help, and the examiner must appreciate and demonstrate his peculiar relationship in his statements and actions.

The recorded history should be pertinent to the problem and not an accumulation of routine and unrelated facts. To facilitate the history-taking process, the examiner should develop a format or outline. This guide permits an orderly approach but does not take the place of a continuing thought process (Fig. 18-1). Asking the significant questions and recording the important answers in an intelligible manner is difficult and requires a great deal of experience and practice.

Certain patients present the facts in a straightforward manner, and history taking is a pleasure. Other patients either do not answer the question or spend considerable time describing tangential matters that do not bear on the making of the diagnosis. The examiner must exercise patience in this instance and not only restate various questions but clarify the information obtained. The history should be as concise as possible and still contain the relevant material.

The information obtained must not only be recorded in a systematic way but also must be legible. The reason for this is so obvious that the statement will not be expanded.

The following is an outline upon which a satisfactory history may be obtained if associated with patient concern and thoughtful consideration.

GENERAL INFORMATION

Certain routine information should be recorded on every patient not only to identify him but also to gain insight into his environmental situation. The patient's name, age, sex, and marital status are essential. The residential address and telephone are important for subsequent contact with the patient. Determining and recording the patient's nationality, occupation, and employer permits the examiner to communicate with the patient and demonstrate interest in him. These areas may be expanded if relevant to the medical problem.

HISTORY

The questions and records are divided into specific categories to ensure that all the pertinent facts are obtained. The medical information overlaps in some areas, but the examiner must organize the material into a concise presentation, deleting repetition.

Chief complaint

The chief complaint is a brief statement describing the patient's presenting symptom or symptoms as well as their duration. The chief complaint indicates the reason why the patient sought medical help and is the focal point for the other parts of the history. The complaint should be recorded succinctly and, if appropriate, in the patient's own words.

Present illness

The present illness develops the chief complaint and describes the illness or injury in chronologic order. Any facts relating to the medical problem should be included in this section.

ONSET. The exact time and manner of onset of symptoms must be established. The hour, day, and month as well as the patient's activity at this time should be recorded. The rapidity with which the symptoms appeared should be indicated, as well as any associated constitutional complaints, for example, fever or chills. If the symptoms are the result of an accident, the mechanism of injury should be determined. The record must reflect how, why, and where the injury occurred; whether the patient was working or not; the direction and magnitude of forces involved; and the immediate disability suffered by the patient. If there has been an injury, the patient should always be asked if he lost consciousness and for what period of time.

After the type and exact location of the presenting symptoms are determined, the patient should be specifically asked whether there are additional related complaints.

COURSE PRIOR TO MEDICAL EVALUATION. The course of the medical problem prior to seeking medical attention must be developed. Relevant information would include a change in symptoms (better or worse) and the appearance of any new symptoms. The patient's activity after the onset should be noted, as well as the success or failure of any medicines or home remedies tried. If some time has elapsed since the symptoms began, the exact reason for the patient seeking medical help at this time should be determined. What change brought the patient to the examiner? On-the-job injuries are routinely reported to the employer, and the history should state whether this procedure has been followed. If the patient has been unable to work, the onset and length of disability should be noted.

The mode of patient's transportation—for instance, car or ambulance—may be pertinent.

PRIOR MEDICAL CARE. The patient should be asked if he has received prior medical care. The physician rendering care, the time, and the reason for changing doctors should be determined. The type of evaluation including diagnostic studies and the results are pertinent. The treatment rendered should be developed as to type and benefits. Any untoward incidents such as allergic reactions or increased symptoms must be recorded.

All previous hospitalizations for the present illness must be described. This information should include the date and length of hospitalization, diagnostic procedures performed, conservative and operative treatment rendered, and the results. Any complications associated with the hospitalization should be developed for cause.

Often the patient will have been seen by a number of physicians, and these visits must all be recorded. The date of the last medical care in relation to the present evaluation is important.

This part of the record should indicate the patient's general activities during this interval. What was the disability? Was he working?

Present symptoms

This section develops in detail the patient's immediate symptom complex. The complaints include those at the time of examination as well as those in the preceding hours or days precipitating medical evaluation. Each symptom must be thoroughly investigated to determine the course.

Symptoms are subjective and quite variable. The list is long, but those symptoms most important to the orthopaedist are pain, numbness, weakness, and loss of function. These symptoms as well as any others must be evaluated by the following criteria. These guidelines are not inclusive and represent only the start.

LOCATION AND RADIATION. The exact location of pain or numbness and radiation of these symptoms must be established.

CHARACTER. The severity and quality of weakness and pain should be described. In the latter instance, is the pain sharp, aching, burning, other?

ASSOCIATED SYMPTOMS. Loss of joint function is often associated with limitation of motion, swelling, and pain. Whatever the primary complaint, it should be related to the entire symptom complex.

WHAT MAKES IT WORSE? The activities or position of the patient, the time of day, or the weather may increase the present symptoms.

WHAT MAKES IT BETTER? Medications, heat, or cold often relieve the discomfort or disability.

EXTENT OF DISABILITY. The degree to which the symptoms restrict the patient's activities must be determined. The reasons for the limitation should be developed.

COURSE. Symptoms are rarely stationary, and a specific statement pertaining to their improvement or worsening is important. Occasionally the complaints are unchanged for a prolonged interval; this is relevant.

Past history

The past history records information pertaining to the patient's previous medical problems. These facts usually do not assist in making the correct diagnosis for the present difficulties but are essential if treatment is to be rendered.

GENERAL HEALTH. The patient should be asked a broad question about his general health. This may bring forth a few or many prior difficulties. Each problem must be recorded including diagnosis, treatment, and present condition.

SERIOUS ILLNESSES. Any significant medical problems should be recorded, noting particularly the diagnosis, treatment, and residual disability. Medications received and any untoward response are pertinent.

SERIOUS INJURIES. Previous trauma must be listed, with particular emphasis on the residuals at the time of onset of the present medical problem. Important information overlooked in the present illness may come to light.

OPERATIONS. The patient's previous surgeries should be listed chronologically, once more determining the diagnosis, reason for surgery, and sequelae. Of particular importance is a description of any postoperative complication.

MEDICATIONS. A list of current medications and the condition being treated should be recorded.

ALLERGIES. The patient must be asked if he is allergic to any drugs or materials. If the answer is affirmative, the type of reaction and sequelae should be developed.

Social history

This portion of the history has no rigid requirements. However, it affords the examiner the opportunity to gain insight into the patient's life style. Questions pertaining to specific areas such as smoking habits or drinking abuses are secondary. More pertinent are the patient's previous and present vocations, avocations, and expectations. Some knowledge of the patient's home life and close personal relationships is often invaluable. Questions pertaining to birthplace and subsequent places of residence demonstrate an interest in the patient as a person. If the patient has been in the military, his branch of service, assignments, and experiences as well as type of discharge are worth exploring.

The questions asked should permit the examiner insight into the patient's social situation without the appearance of prying into his personal affairs. The interview should increase rapport and not diminish it.

Family history

This section of the history should be brief. Any history of recurring medical problems in the patient's family should be determined. Of particular interest is a family history of diabetes, anemia, or infectious disease.

Any medical conditions in the patient's present illness or past history should be explored for a possible family or hereditary relationship.

CHAPTER 19

ORTHOPAEDIC EXAMINATION

GENERAL CONSIDERATIONS

A description of a detailed general physical examination is beyond the scope of this presentation. The material will be limited to certain routine observations and measurements necessary in an orthopaedic specialty examination to determine the diagnosis, follow the patient's progress, and evaluate permanent disability.

SUBJECTIVE VERSUS OBJECTIVE OBSERVATION

Subjective physical findings are under the voluntary control of the patient. Tenderness to palpation, muscle weakness, numbness, and limitation of joint motion are in this category. These disabilities may be caused by organic pathology; however, in each instance they are under the voluntary control of the patient and may be feigned. Subjective findings are extremely important but must be carefully evaluated (Fig. 19-1).

Objective observations are measurable and reproducible. Limb lengths and circumferences, size and shape of tumors, signs of redness, and heat are objective. Mensuration must be deliberate and accurate. The measurements should be repeated as necessary to make sure the findings are reliable.

EXAMINATION

General appearance

On the basis of his appearance, the examiner should determine and record the patient's general state of health, nutrition, and discomfort. Is he healthy and well developed or acutely or chronically ill? Is he slender or obese? Does he appear in acute distress or seem relatively comfortable? This superficial appraisal assists in the evaluation of the potential urgency of the problem.

The patient's reaction to the interview and examination is significant. Is he cooperative, anxious, reticent, or vague? The record must reflect only the examiner's observations and not his diagnostic impressions. If a patient presents with slurred speech and an alcoholic breath, these facts

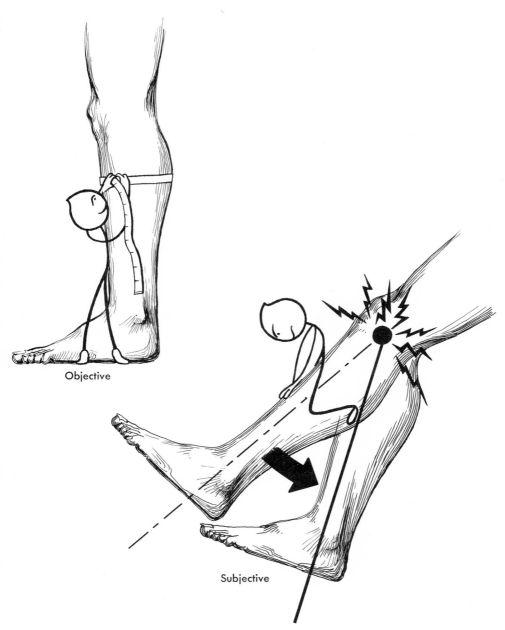

Objective

Subjective

Fig. 19-1. Subjective versus objective.

should be noted; however, a statement indicating alcoholic intoxication must not be made. This diagnosis is premature and may be incorrect. Later review of such a statement leads to unfortunate consequences. Objective observation and reporting are the important requirements.

Gait and body mobility

The patient's gait and general mobility should be observed and recorded. Careful scrutiny of a limp is necessary to distinguish among various causes. An abnormal gait may result from pain, muscular weakness, or a short leg; however, the differentiation is often difficult. The patient's need for crutches or a cane should be noted.

The ease and rapidity with which a patient gets in and out of a chair, on and off an examining table, or dresses and undresses himself are significant in determining disability. The patient occasionally performs better when he is not being directly observed. Any unusual body position or motion is recorded objectively without an associated diagnostic impression.

Cervical, thoracic, and lumbar spines

A large proportion of orthopaedic office practice deals with acute, subacute, and chronic conditions of the spine. Although spinal pathology is diverse and complex, the pertinent local physical findings described by inspection, palpation, and the determination of spinal motion are usually sufficient to evaluate the problem in conjunction with an examination of the upper and lower extremities.

The examiner should be familiar with the normal anatomy and mobility of the three areas of the spine. The normal not only varies between patients but alters with age. Experience is required to recognize and evaluate the abnormal; however, accurate objective observation is still possible without it.

CERVICAL SPINE

Inspection. The normal cervical spine demonstrates a gentle lordotic curve without scoliosis. Alteration of the curve or a torticollis should be described as to extent and position.

Palpation. Palpation must always be gentle, but the amount of pressure required to produce pain is important. The tenderness elicited may be well localized or diffuse and reproducible or not. Careful inspection of the area for associated redness, heat, or swelling is pertinent. The determination of muscle spasm or tightness by touch is not reliable.

Motion. Spinal motion, whether in the cervical, thoracic, or lumbar areas, should always be voluntary. Additional information is not gained by forced passive motion, but patient discomfort is increased with possible hazards.

Cervical spine motion may be recorded as follows:

1. **Flexion:** The distance in inches the chin lacks touching the sternum
2. **Extension:** The distance in inches the occipital prominence lacks touching the most prominent spinous process (C7 or T1)
3 and 4. **Right and left rotation:** The angle in degrees the nose makes to the sagittal plane of the body
5 and 6. **Right and left lateral bend:** The angle in degrees the head makes with the trunk in the sagittal plane

Any pain elicited during these maneuvers should be described for location and intensity. The patient should be asked whether pain limits the motion.

THORACIC SPINE. The thoracic spine has a gentle kyphosis without gibbus or scoliosis. The shoulders and scapulae are level. The thoracic spine has no significant motion that can be recorded; however, chest excursion with inspiration and aspiration may be of significance.

The examination should describe any variance from normal by inspection and palpation. The circumferential measurements of the chest at the nipple line in inspiration and aspiration are recorded.

LUMBAR SPINE

Inspection. The lumbar spine has a mild lordosis that is normally accentuated in pregnant women and abdominal obesity. The lordosis is usually somewhat decreased in older patients. With the patient standing, the iliac crests should be at the same level. A difference in the two heights suggests a scoliosis or leg length discrepancy. The record should indicate any lumbar flattening or list.

Palpation. Points and areas of tenderness elicited by palpation should be inspected for local cause. The degree of pressure required to produce the pain should be noted as well as the consistency of the location.

Motion. Lumbar spine motion is recorded as follows:

1. **Flexion:** The distance in inches the fingertips lack touching the floor with the knees extended. Flexion normally reverses the lordotic curve and is smooth. Failure to flatten the curve or jerkiness should be noted.
2. **Extension:** The percentage of the normal voluntary arc of motion for this patient
3 and 4. **Right and left lateral bend:** The percentage of the normal voluntary arc of motion for this patient
5 and 6. **Right and left rotation:** The percentage of the normal voluntary arc of motion for this patient. Associated with these maneuvers are pain and limitation of motion secondary to discomfort. These should be described as to location, severity, and duration (Fig. 19-2).

Limb lengths

The accurate determination of limb lengths requires measurement between two bony prominences with the extremities in similar positions. The findings are recorded as right over left or injured over uninjured side.

UPPER EXTREMITIES. The length of the upper extremities is measured from

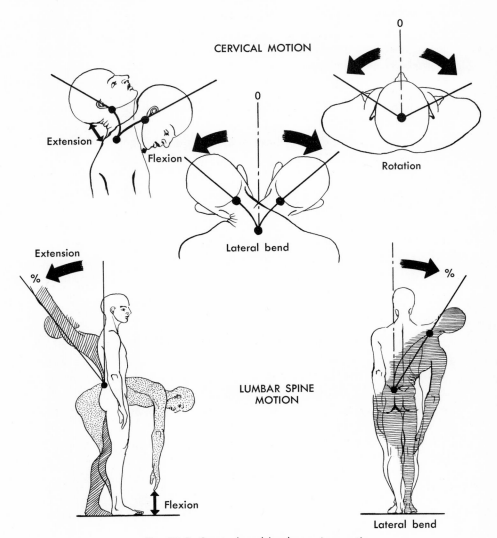

Fig. 19-2. Cervical and lumbar spine motion.

the tip of the acromion process to the radial styloid. The patient is erect with the upper extremities hanging freely to the side, the elbows in extension, and the forearms in supination. The bony prominences are accurately localized, and the tape is fixed proximally to the acromion and run distally over the lateral arm and forearm to the radial styloid. The measurements are recorded as previously described. The major side or dominant hand must be indicated.

LOWER EXTREMITIES. True leg lengths are measured from the anterior superior iliac spines to the medial malleoli. The former bony prominence may be difficult to localize exactly because of fatty subcutaneous tissue or an overlying pendulous abdomen, and repetitive palpation may be necessary to determine the precise area. The measurement is carried out with the patient supine and the knees extended. After identifying the anterior superior iliac spine, the tape is placed just distal to it, engaging the notch, and down the leg to the medial malleolus. Considerable practice is necessary to record reproducible results.

Limb circumferences

Limb circumference measurements must be performed at the same level on both sides to be of value. In general, limbs are measured at their maximum girth; however, "eye balling" the site is unreliable. Both extremities should be marked a specific distance from a bony prominence as determined by a tape. The exact distances from the prominences is not so important as the fact that they are the same.

The muscles must be relaxed for accurate measurements. The tape is placed snugly about the limb with the touching sides adjacent and parallel to the skin mark. The tension applied to the tape must be the same on both sides for satisfactory comparison (Fig. 19-3).

ARM CIRCUMFERENCE. Arm circumference is measured 7 to 9 inches from the bony tip of the acromion down the midlateral arm. The patient is sitting or standing with the upper extremities relaxed and hanging to the side.

FOREARM CIRCUMFERENCE. Forearm circumference is measured 3 to 4 inches distal to the medial epicondyle of the humerus. The patient is seated with the forearms in supination and resting on the anterior thighs and the elbows in the equal amounts of flexion. The volar forearms are marked transversely at the correct levels and mensuration is carried out.

THIGH CIRCUMFERENCE. Thigh circumference is measured 8 to 10 inches proximal to the adductor tubercle of the femur. The patient is supine with muscles relaxed and the knee extended.

Mensuration can be performed using the superior border of the patella as the identifying bony prominence; however, this is not a fixed point and will not be as accurate.

LEG CIRCUMFERENCE. Leg circumference is performed 2 to 4 inches distal to the bony prominence with the patient supine and the knee extended.

Joint motion

GENERAL CONSIDERATIONS. There has been confusion in recording joint motion in the past because "neutral" or "anatomic" position has been described by different numbers of degrees. The American Academy of Orthopaedic Surgeons has adopted the terminology in which the "neutral" position of any joint is 0 degrees and flexion, extension, abduction, and so on are measured from this starting point. The extended knee

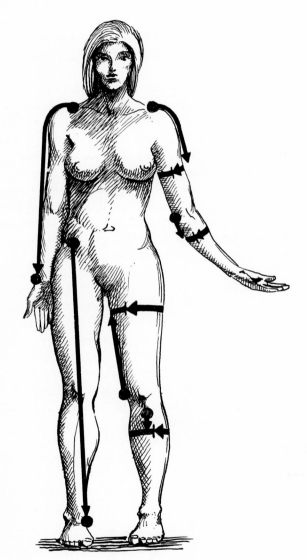

Fig. 19-3. Mensuration.

and elbow were previously recorded as 180 degrees; however, this "neutral" or "anatomic" position of these joints is now 0 degrees. If either of these joints exceeds 0 degrees, the position is termed "hyperextension" and not "extension." Lack of complete extension in the elbow and knee is described as a "flexion deformity."

Joint motions are measured with a goniometer. The two limbs of this instrument are placed in line with the bones on each side of the joint and with its center over the axis of motion. The position of the joint in number of degrees is then read off the goniometer. The use of the goniometer is made difficult if the bones on each side of a joint are obscured by muscle mass. However, with practice and patience reproducible readings can be obtained.

RECORDING JOINT MOTION. Joint motion is recorded as right over left or or injured over uninjured, either in degrees or in percentages.

ACTIVE VERSUS PASSIVE. Joint motions are recorded as active or passive. Active motion measures the joint range of motion performed voluntarily by the patient. Passive motion measures the amount of joint motion possible by the examiner's manipulation. The latter maneuver must be cautious and, if any pain is elicited, should be immediately stopped.

SHOULDER JOINT MOTION. The shoulder joint is considered to be in neutral or 0 position with the arm against the chest, the elbow extended, and the forearm in neutral position.

Joint measurements

abduction Angle in degrees between arm and trunk in lateral sagittal plane
adduction Angle between arm and trunk in medial sagittal plane
flexion Angle in degrees between arm and trunk in anterior coronal plane
extension Angle in degrees between arm and trunk in posterior coronal plane
internal rotation° Angle in degrees between forearm and horizontal in internal rotation
external rotation° Angle in degrees between forearm and horizontal in external rotation

ELBOW JOINT MOTION. Neutral position or 0 degrees occurs when the arm and forearm are in a straight line (Fig. 19-4).

Joint measurements

flexion Angle in degrees between arm and forearm with elbow bent completely
flexion deformity Angle in degrees between arm and forearm with elbow extended
hyperextension Angle in degrees between arm and forearm beyond a straight line

FOREARM JOINT MOTION. Neutral position for the forearm is measured with the arms to the patient's side, the elbow flexed to 90 degrees, and the forearms in a position of midrotation, namely, with the thumbs up.

°This measurement is carried out with the patient standing and the arms abducted to 90 degrees in neutral flexion and extension and the elbow flexed to 90 degrees.

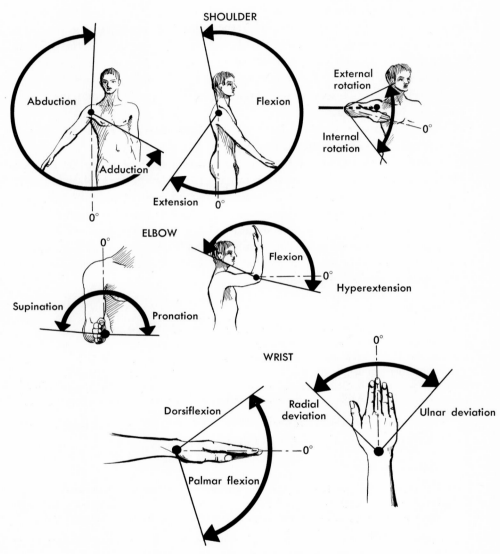

Fig. 19-4. Joint motion: upper extremity.

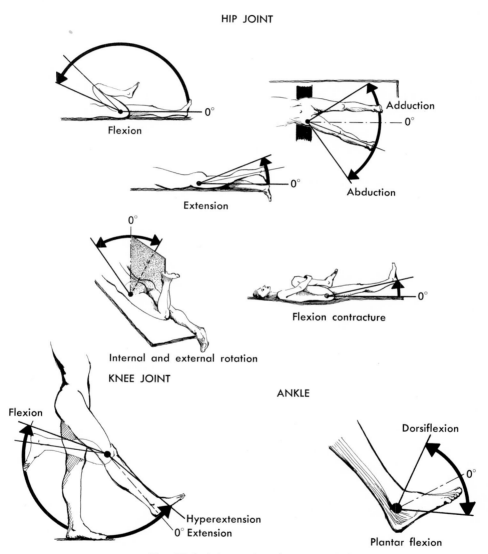

Fig. 19-5. Joint motion: lower extremity.

Joint measurements

pronation Angle in degrees between palm and horizontal in pronation
supination Angle in degrees between palm and horizontal in supination

WRIST JOINT MOTION. Neutral position or 0 degrees of the wrist joint is with the radius and long finger metacarpal in a straight line in all planes.

Joint measurements

dorsiflexion Angle in degrees between forearm and metacarpals in extension
palmar flexion Angle in degrees between forearm and metacarpals in flexion
ulnar deviation Angle in degrees between long finger metacarpal and forearm in ulnar deviation
radial deviation Angle in degrees between long finger metacarpal and forearm in radial deviation

HIP JOINT MOTION. The 0 position of the hip joint aligns the thigh with the trunk in all planes. Most measurements are performed with the patient supine or prone.

Joint measurements

flexion Angle in degrees between trunk and thigh in anterior sagittal plane
extension Angle in degrees between trunk and thigh in posterior sagittal plane
abduction Angle in degrees between trunk and thigh in lateral coronal plane
internal rotation* Angle in degrees between leg and vertical in internal rotation
external rotation* Angle in degrees between leg and vertical in external rotation
flexion contracture Angle in degrees that the thigh lacks in alignment with lumbar spine flexed (accomplished with the patient supine and completely flexing the opposite hip (Fig. 19-5)

KNEE JOINT MOTION. Neutral or 0 degrees occurs with the thigh and legs in a straight line.

Joint measurements

flexion Angle in degrees between thigh and leg with knee completely bent
flexion deformity Angle in degrees between thigh and leg with knee extended
hyperextension Angle in degrees between thigh and leg beyond a straight line

ANKLE JOINT MOTION. Neutral or 0 degrees occurs when the leg and foot are at a right angle.

Joint measurements

plantar flexion Angle in degrees between the leg and foot with the foot in equinus
dorsiflexion Angle in degrees between the leg and foot with the foot dorsiflexed

---

*This measurement is carried out with the patient prone and the knee joint flexed to 90 degrees.

INDEX